DON'T SUGAR COAT IT

THE 21-DAY SUGAR-FREE DIET

SCOTT POWERS

CONTENTS

INTRODUCTION

"Eating crappy food isn't a reward. It's a PUNISHMENT."

— DREW CARY

Food—how we love it and how we need it! Scrumptious donuts, soul-refreshing juices, and so many mouth-watering delicacies, they are all far too tempting to avoid. Whether we take a bite or consume the entire lot, we just can't get enough.

To almost every one of us, food is just food. Some food tastes good while some just doesn't sit well with our taste buds. We need food, and we clearly cannot imagine our lives without it. Take the food away and you take life away.

This, therefore, makes one thing absolutely clear; we need food, regardless if we like it or not. But do we need all of it? As it turns out, no. While food and water may be the life sources for every living thing on the planet, not all ingredients of that food give life. Some of these ingredients are discreetly taking away life, jeopardizing our health, and pushing our luck further than it has ever gone before. Continue to use these components and what we end up with is a world full of problems, literally.

There are many such ingredients that I could go on to list, but none compares to sugar in the destruction caused. Yes, you read that correctly. Sugar is not your friend. It is just like the back-stabbing enemy that hides in plain sight, disguises itself as your friend, and when you are least attentive, it gets you just like Scar in *The Lion King*. You could be hanging on for dear life, and it will stare at you, smiling and knowing that it has done its job.

We are no strangers to the devastating results sugar can deliver, and some of us might even be experiencing these now. However, even after knowing the facts, we still decided to continue down the path that leads to certain doom. Over 25,000 Americans lose their lives each year just from consuming sugar consumption, and that is not even scratching the surface. In total, 180,000 people lose their lives every year worldwide due to sugar (Healy, 2015).

I do not wish to alarm you, or at least not yet, but it takes only one good look around you to know that things are clearly going wrong, and if anything is to be blamed, it is sugar.

In 1962, over half a century ago, 46% of American adults were considered either overweight or obese. A staggering number, isn't it? It gets worse. In 2010, that number sky-rocketed and encompassed 75% of American adults, and that was a decade ago (Johns Hopkins Medicine, n.d.). This unprecedented leap in overweight and obesity numbers has gone on to change the landscape completely and has forced all of us to rethink what we think is good food.

If that wasn't enough, the real damage was reported by Reuters in 2017. They reported that a jaw-dropping 11 million people died in 2017 alone worldwide, from deaths related to poor diets that included "high sugar, salt, and processed meat" (Kelland, 2019). All of these components contribute to heart disease, cancers, diabetes, and other ailments, the same study found. The nail in the coffin comes in the fact that these are the deaths that were reported and studied, meaning there were many others throughout the world who have died related deaths but were never added into the report.

Consume too much sugar, and it consumes you in return. I wish there was a better way to put this, but throughout my years in the medical field, I have observed firsthand the devastation that sugar brings to everyone. For years, I have met people who just cannot resist the temptations of indulging in food with a high sugar content. When advised that there are better alternatives with no sugar, they quickly frown and dismiss the entire idea of "tasteless food."

What people fail to realize is that if they just put their mind to it, they can prepare some of the most delicious and scrumptious meals they have ever tasted without the use of sugar. The idea may seem strange, but it is achievable, it is possible, and by the end of this book, it is all yours to enjoy for the rest of your life. All I ask is patience, perseverance, and 21 consecutive days of your life. Sounds like a lot, I know, but it will soon pass, and before you know it, you will be enjoying some of the most tasteful recipes and possibly teaching others how they can do the same as well. A healthier alternative is what awaits everyone at the end of this book.

Both you and I will see to it that we learn all we can about just how destructive sugar can be, how we can learn to avoid the temptation, and how a sugar-free diet benefits us in the long run. Of course, this is only the first half of the book. The second half of the book will take you through what really interests you, the recipes.

To make things easier, I have ensured that this book does not contain many complex, hard-to-understand terms. If used, they are only done so to facilitate the learning experience. I will do all I can to ensure that these terms, wherever they are used, are clearly explained. My intention is not to confuse you but to provide you with knowledge that is helpful and can help you make the necessary changes to lead a better life.

WHO SHOULD READ THIS BOOK?

Ah, that is a valid question. Not all books are meant for everyone to read, but since we are talking about life itself, and how to live it better, it applies to everyone who is at least 18 years old or above.

Whether you are an underweight woman, aged 35, or a man slightly tipping the scales above the red line, just 18 years of age, this book offers information that suits any adult at any age.

I intend to address everyone who has been struggling or facing adverse health effects from consumption of sugar, I will provide you with all the necessary information, recipes, and tips to ensure that you can have something to look forward to every day. No longer will you need to worry about your sugar intake, and with a peaceful mind, you will be able to enjoy life at its finest, without any sign of sugar in sight.

If you are someone who is overweight, or obese for that matter, do not worry. I do not claim that you will lose weight instantly, or that you will take a certain period of time to see any results, but what I do assure you is that you will enjoy these healthier alternatives. Eventually, the benefits this "no-sugar" diet will bring you will be evident, and you will go on to lead a better life. I have seen many whom I have helped, and the results only fill me up with confidence.

In addition, I cannot forget people who may be like me, who are neither overweight nor suffering adverse health effects. These are the people who have seen the devastation firsthand or read far too much about it and want to ensure that they do not also fall victim. Your timing couldn't be any better. Those who start early and steer clear of such things are bound to gain the most significant results of all. Now is better than tomorrow, and we all know that tomorrow is the excuse that never dies.

Sugar is bad, and I cannot stress this point enough. Throughout the first part of this book, through Chapter 4, you will learn just how dangerous it is to consume too much sugar. You will also come to learn the extent of the damage sugar has done to the world through the years.

"Wait, why do I wanna learn about the damage? Why not jump straight to the good bit?"

To overcome something, one must first learn all about it. As the famous quote goes:

"Knowing is half the battle."

— UNKNOWN

This is true for every situation in life. The more you increase your knowledge about something, the better the results will be for you because you will know reactions to a certain action, or what can happen if something changes. Without knowledge, we are just like sailboats lost at sea, without the ability to steer, navigate, or even communicate. We are at the mercy of the sea to slosh us from side to side, hoping that we will eventually arrive somewhere safe. That somewhere will rarely come, and even if it does, it may no longer mean anything to us.

This book will provide you with:

- An in-depth understanding of sugar and how it harms us
- Methods to overcome sugar cravings
- A properly laid out 21-day sugar-free plan to get you in the groove
- All the tools you need to become autonomous after the 21-day period, to continue your newly adopted sugar-free life
- Plenty of useful information to lead a healthier life

These are just some of the things you will come across. A lot awaits us ahead, and with that being said, let me quickly address the obvious elephant in the room.

Who Am I?

Whenever we pick up a book, we have this natural instinct to learn who the author is. When it comes to self-help books or cookbooks, we really need to know who we are following; that is a natural concern.

My name is Scott Powers. I am a nurse, with over a decade of experience treating so many patients, including diabetics. I have seen the devastation firsthand, and I have used my experience to put together tips and tricks to help those around me to avoid these perils. I am happily married, and I have two kids, which means that I am far too conscious about the type of food that enters my home.

For years, I have tried to learn all I can about a good sugar-free diet. I have tried many and found that most had no idea what they were talking about. As a nurse, I hold an edge because I know the type of things which are present in these so-called "diets" that people often advertise.

This pursuit led me to start experimenting with food and learn the best possible ways to avoid sugar in my food. Since I am fond of reading and cooking, things were somewhat easier but figuring out what the better options were did take time. Fortunately, after much trial and error, I found what I was looking for.

My days of being a nurse were over as I found my calling. I found a way through which I could help a lot more people than I normally could. Using my experience as a nurse and the knowledge that comes with it, I decided to help everyone who needed it. Sure enough, my initial method was limiting me to a select few people, and that is why I decided to write a book instead.

Don't Sugar Coat It is my way to give something back to the community, with all clarity and honesty. I intend to debunk all the myths that I have come across so far and expose the truth. I intend to spread awareness to the masses so that they know how they are being manipulated into believing that their food is "safe" to consume.

It is an ambitious mission, to say the least, but it is one that I intend to achieve by the end of this book. The journey is long and arduous, but it is not impossible.

"The journey of a thousand miles begins with one step."

— *LAO TZU*

SUGAR BIAS

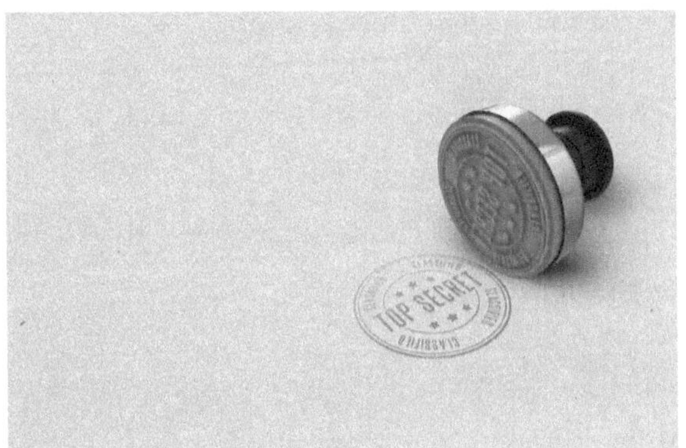

It is somewhat funny to see that despite the repeated warnings and commercials, people still tend to use and consume sugar. There is no denying the fact that we, as human beings, are attracted to sugar just like a moth is attracted to a flame. In both these instances, the source of attraction remains while those attracted are literally consumed in the process.

Almost every other product we pick up has added sugar, and it has now become virtually impossible to find something that does not contain any added sugar elements. Most shopping carts that leave the counter of any superstore on Earth contain a large number of items that have sugary ingredients within them.

The problem lies in the fact that most of the advertisements, blogs, and even books we read continue to push the idea that it is okay to consume sugar, as long as we do not go above a certain limit. If we were to be honest for a moment, we would immediately know that most of us do not keep track of how much sugar we have consumed today, or the day before, or how much we need to consume the day after.

The other problem comes in the fact that if sugar is as unhealthy as I am trying to portray, how come there is a massive abundance of it in the markets? That is a question worth pondering.

We all have our poisons, but sugar is one that is universal. Everyone loves it, everyone thinks they need it, but almost no one has an idea of what sugar exactly is. While we go on to consume it, we never really stop to think how sugar affects our bodies and why some experts continue to say that sugar is bad for our health. This chapter, therefore, is a dose of reality, an eye-opener, and hopefully a comprehensive answer to all such questions. It will highlight exactly what and how harmful sugar is.

THE SCIENCE OF SUGAR

To fully define and understand what sugar is, we must go back to its origins and its structure. Only then will we fully be able to explain to ourselves, and those who may inquire later on, what sugar really is.

Sugar is a simple carbohydrate. A lot of food substances have a general name and a chemical name. While sugar may be the common name, its chemical name is sucrose. I am sure you have come across that name at some point in time, and now you know what it really means.

This chemical is produced naturally within all plants, including but not limited to vegetables, nuts, and fruits. Of course, since we are talking about plants, the term photosynthesis comes to mind. This is the natural process through which plants receive sunlight and absorb CO_2, and, well, all of us know the rest. What our science teachers failed to mention was the part where sucrose is created during this process.

As plants go on to pull minerals and water from the ground, the leaves, at the same time, absorb carbon dioxide from the air. This is then followed by chlorophyll (what essentially gives plants and leaves their green color) absorbing energy directly from the sun. This energy is absorbed within the leaf cells.

At this point, the plant now has water and minerals, which it pulled from the ground through its roots, and carbon dioxide.

This means the plant is now ready to process these into something called sucrose. It does so by using the sun's energy, carbon dioxide, and water, which ends up creating sucrose that is then stored within these plants.

Of course, not all plants have the same capacities for holding sucrose. There are some plants which have lower quantities of it, while there are some which tend to hold higher sucrose values. When it comes to the latter, sugar beets and the mighty sugar cane take the prize. These two plants store the highest quantity of sugar, which is why they are naturally selected as the source to extract sugar from.

Now comes the interesting bit. The sugar that is extracted from these two ideal sources is exactly the same as the one you eat when consuming fruits or nuts. It is in its purest form, all natural, and has no hint of additives or preservatives. Of course, this may come as a bit of good news to some of us because the sugar we normally store within our pantries is exactly the same.

So far, quite simple to understand. However, we cannot just stop there and think "Ah, now I know what sugar is." The fact is that sugar is a little more complicated than that. To fully explain that, I will need to act as a chemistry teacher, so bear with me as students.

We know that sugar is sucrose and vice-versa. However, on a microscopic level, things seem to be different. The simple chemical structure of sugar itself is rather simple. It is just a single molecule of glucose, bonded together with another molecule of fructose, and we have mother nature to thank for that bond.

"Glucose, and fructose. Sounds delicious."

They most certainly tend to be, and that is because these two are also a form of sugar. If we break sugar down, we will end up with three simple sugars, each of which is called a monosaccharide.

A monosaccharide is nothing more than a single or one-molecule sugar. Since we are talking about sugar, there are three monosaccharides found within plants and other sources of sugar. These go on to bond with each other easily to create more complex carbohydrates, the types of which I will not go into exact details of as that would only be confusing.

All of the carbohydrates you can think of are made of at least one molecule of sugar, or more. When these carbohydrates are consumed within our bodies, regardless of their complexities, they are all broken down into their simpler forms: glucose, galactose, and fructose.

I would not be wrong to say that they are considered as "building blocks" which go on to make up all kinds of carbohydrates.

"Wait, I count two, not three."

The three monosaccharides, or simple sugars, are:

- Glucose - This is virtually in every food.
- Fructose - Mostly found in fruits.
- Galactose - This is found in milk.

To give you an idea of the kind of bonds and complex carbohydrates these go on to make, here is a list that showcases what these three monosaccharides can make when they bond with each other:

Disaccharides (when two monosaccharides combine)

- Sucrose (also known as table sugar) – Glucose combined with fructose
- Lactose (Milk sugar) – Glucose combined with galactose
- Maltose (Malt sugar) – Glucose combined with glucose

Polysaccharides (When more than 10 monosaccharides combine together)

- Starch – This is a glucose polymer, meaning that more than 10 glucose molecules combine and bond together. Starch is what plants use to store any excess glucose for later use.

Now, the eagle-eyed reader may have spotted that glucose was common in each of these bonds, and there is a perfectly logical reason behind that. Carbohydrates are the go-to source of energy for our bodies, not because they taste good, but because they contain glucose. Just as jet fuel is the only source of fuel for jet planes, glucose is the only fuel our brain, organs, and all the muscles need to work. Take glucose away from our body, and we would collapse in an instant.

This is exactly why those little devices that poke your finger and collect a droplet of your blood to give a reading are called glucometers. They calculate the amount of glucose present within the blood. If that number goes high, you are in trouble, and if that number goes low, you face more severe issues.

"So, what you are saying is that sugar is nothing more than a carbohydrate?"

In a nutshell, yes. You are right on target with that one. Carbohydrates are our source of fuel for the body. These, along with proteins and fats, are called macronutrients, and they do exactly what they sound like—provide the body with energy to carry out functions.

Is Sugar Fuel?

This may sound a little confusing, but despite being told repeatedly that sugar is bad, we actually need it to stay alive. It is considered as the building block upon which our survival depends.

While we learned how our bodies and brain need this as fuel, what we didn't look into was how this all works.

When we consume fruits or vegetables, we are consuming all the starch these plants once held within themselves. Our body has a natural capability of breaking down the starches and creating glucose out of them. As that happens, our body starts to replenish its supply of glucose and ensures speedy delivery of it to various parts of the body. Of course, we do not know how much starch we should consume at any given time of the day, and that means we can often end up consuming more starch than needed.

Every bit of the excess is broken down into glucose. Our body takes away what it needs and converts the rest into a similar complex sugar called glycogen. This is then stored within our livers for later use.

This brings us to yet another question. Since we have carbohydrates, proteins, and fats that act as fuel, where do we get them from? Let us first learn of the source. Later, we will look into how each of these are also broken down into glucose.

Carbohydrates (the main source of energy)

- bread
- pasta
- potatoes
- rice

- fruit
- vegetables
- sugar
- milk
- yogurt

Our bodies can convert all of the carbohydrates we consume into glucose. This means that once our body is done doing that, our sugar levels are affected in a matter of one to two hours.

Protein

- cheese
- meat
- fish
- peanut butter

Proteins, unlike carbohydrates, are not completely broken down into glucose. Even though our body changes some of the proteins into glucose, most of the glucose is stored away in our livers. This glucose is not released into our bloodstream, meaning that it does not impact or affect our blood sugar levels significantly at all.

Fat

- salad dressing
- butter
- olive oil
- avocado (Kaiser Permanente, 2019)

Our bodies turn less than 10% of the fat we consume into glucose. This glucose, which our body obtains from the fats, is absorbed ever so slowly. There is no immediate rise in our blood sugar levels either.

The point which should be noticed here is the fact that if we were to consume a high-fat meal, it would significantly slow down the carbohydrate digestion process, and this would result in elevated levels of blood sugar in just a few hours after the meal.

This delayed action is usually why people often go to bed with a normal blood sugar reading and wake up to find that their fasting sugar reading has surpassed the 200 mark. The high fat meal was digested slowly overnight, and hence, increased the presence of sugar within the blood.

With all said and done, the entire "we need sugar to live" statement seems a little questionable. However, before you go on to pass judgement on that, it is worth noticing that we do not need sugar in and of itself to survive; we need a form of it. That part is covered by our body's own ability to break down starch, proteins, fats, and carbohydrates into glucose. We may not even have to consume sweet, sugary food to live either. Whatever we consume contains one of these elements, and for our bodies, that is more than enough to get the process going.

The main question that rises at this point is this:

If our bodies are able to break food down into simple sugar, such as glucose, why do we crave sweet things? Truthfully speaking, this has little to do with a food being "sugary" in nature. The actual reason why that happens is a lot different than the one you might be thinking about.

The Temptations

As soon as we start eating cakes, or cookies, or any sugary food, our body produces a chemical called dopamine. For those who may not know, dopamine is also called as the "feel-good" chemical. When released into our bodies, we instantly feel good and happy. It is effectively our body's way of rewarding ourselves.

Everyone loves to do something that makes them happy over and over again. In a similar fashion, our body also wants to do something over and over again, just so it can feel good. What you are effectively looking at is addiction coming to life.

Every time we consume sugar, or anything that pushes our body to produce dopamine, our body will force us to do the same action again. This is why when we eat sugary food, our bodies push us to consume more, hence the cravings that kick in every now and then.

Our brain is wired to do so many things. It decides what kind of food it likes and what it doesn't. Since we have evolved from our primitive selves, it is easy to see why we have come to love sweet foods and find them that much more pleasurable. Rewind the clock thousands of years, and we were nothing more than scavengers. They relied on these sugary foods to give them the energy they needed to survive. This love affair with sweet food was imprinted in their personalities, and thousands of years later, we are still experiencing the same pleasure.

Our brain's reward system, when activated, fires dopamine, and that goes on to alter our behavior, and we already know how this makes it more likely that we will do the same thing again. Considering the fact that we are surrounded by a variety of sweet options, it is rather easy for us to fall for one, and that is where the trouble starts.

If we were to cave into our body's demand for sweets, our mind will eventually be rewired through a process called neuroplasticity. This process does not necessarily happen only when the reward system kicks in, but we will only be focusing on that for now. If we were to continue consuming more sugary foods, our mind would start creating a tolerance.

When tolerance is created, we stop feeling good by consuming the same amount of sweet foods. Now, to feel the reward system kick back in, we need to eat more. Continue that for a while and a new tolerance level is created, and the process just keeps on going until you are quite literally a sugar addict.

Addiction 101

Addiction of any kind follows the same process. It activates our reward system, which produces dopamine, which then makes us feel good. After a while, the tolerance levels build up, and we are forced to do more of what we did before, just to feel good again. In the case of sugar, however, there is a long debate that has been going on for ages. There are those who claim that this isn't even a real thing, and then there are those who continue to support the idea of sugar addiction being a reality.

Sugar can indeed cause addiction, and it is similar to cocaine addiction. There are many signs through which you can find out if you, or someone else, has sugar addiction. Some of these are:

- You are not comfortable sharing with anyone the fact that you eat sugar.
- You eat sugar, even though you may not be feeling hungry.
- You feel satisfied when you consume sugar.
- You constantly find yourself craving sugary food.
- You also crave salty foods.
- If you try to quit, you end up with unusual symptoms.

- When stressed or anxious, you use sugary food to calm yourself.
- Despite knowing the consequences, you consume sugar anyway.
- You often go out of your way just to get sugar.
- You feel guilty for consuming sugar.

These are some classical signs that all point at you, or someone else, being a sugar addict. If you are an addict, it is high time to seek help, and hopefully, stop in time before any serious or irreparable damage is done to the body.

How Does a Sugar-Free Diet Work?

No diet can ever be 100% sugar free. There are always carbohydrates in every meal we consume, and we already know that carbohydrates are later broken into simple sugar forms. Now, if we cannot avoid it, what can we do? Well, our aim is to avoid any added or excess sugar, and that is where we have a world full of options to explore.

Dr. Kristina Rother of the National Institute of Health says, "Glucose is the number one food for the brain, and it's an extremely important source of fuel throughout the body." She then says, "But there's no need to add glucose to your diet, because your body can make the glucose it needs by breaking down food molecules like carbohydrates, proteins, and fats" (National Institute of Health, 2014).

This is possibly the best explanation you can come across at this point in time. While our body needs the glucose to work, it is completely unnecessary for us to add additional glucose as our body has the ability to break down carbohydrates, proteins, and fats into the glucose it needs to work.

There is another good reason why one should not be putting any added sugar into foods. Generally, fructose and sucrose are the two forms of sugar we add to our food items. These are known to have something called "empty calories," which essentially means that they contain no nutritional value.

"If that is the case, why bother avoiding it?"

Although they do not provide any upside to us, if they are consumed, there is, however, massive downside to these empty calories. A number of researchers have found that excess sugar can lead a person to develop liver toxicity and a number of other chronic diseases, including Alzheimer's. Added sugar is known to cause many other chronic conditions, all of which can prove to be fatal if left unattended or unchecked.

The Wolf in Sheep's Clothing

Unlike it's sibling monosaccharide glucose, fructose is processed only by the liver. No other body part is able to process fructose. How does that put us in any danger, you might ask? By consuming larger quantities of fructose, one can develop nonalcoholic fatty liver disease, which eventually leads to liver failure and death.

This means that despite the claims of fructose being a "friendly" form of sugar, it is dangerous when consumed in excess amounts, and it is something we must all learn to steer clear of, or at least avoid as much as possible.

Now, I did mention that fructose comes naturally, and that means it is also present in some of our favorite fruits as well. Does that mean we should start avoiding them? Absolutely not. The fructose present within these fruits is not enough to cause any kind of harm to a human body. Our liver can easily process the natural, unprocessed form of fructose found within all-natural fruits, and that is because we also consume fiber in the process. Fiber is known to facilitate the digestion process, meaning that our body gets the extra help it needs to ensure complete digestion.

Not-so-natural fructose can be found in juices or soda drinks, and these are generally labeled as fiber free. These are the ones to watch out for.

Natural vs. Processed Sugar

Processed sugar is a bit different from natural sugar. It is extracted from sugar canes or sugar beets. It is then processed and treated with various chemicals, including high-fructose corn syrups, before being packed and sold to consumers. When consumed, our bodies rapidly break this type of sugar down, and as a result, our blood sugar levels skyrocket.

Since such food sources are digested quickly, you will not feel full, even if you had a significant quantity of it. This will naturally push you to eat more, exposing your body to risks of developing obesity, and eventually, a higher risk of cancer.

The good news is that it is fairly easy to learn how to reduce the use of processed sugar in your daily life. You can start working on some of these right away. They include, but are not limited to:

- Water – Do not consume energy drinks, sodas, sport drinks, or any other fruit drinks as they comprise around 44% of the added sugar in your diet (Health Designs, 2017).
- Your sauces and toppings – Although we will learn some incredible recipes, it is generally a good idea to try and avoid ketchup, salad dressings, barbeque sauces, and any other condiment that you may find in the market. A better alternative is to rely on fresh herbs, lime, and homemade salad dressings.
- Processed snacks – This may come to you as a bit of a surprise, but even snacks which claim that they are "all natural" or "organic" are brimming with added sugar. A better alternative would be to snack on a mix of nuts or fresh fruits of your choice.

Sweeteners and Sugar Substitutes

There are some of us who have been advised to replace sugar with some form of sweetener because they are "better for us." The truth is that there is no conclusive research that shows if these are actually beneficial over the long term (Smith, 2019). We are still learning if these are a healthier alternative for us in the long run.

Some of us use these to prepare sugar-free desserts while others use them to sweeten their drinks. Regardless of how we use them, these can go on to affect our microbiome.

Microbiome is a balance of bacteria that is present within our gut. It is essential for this balance to remain intact as these special bacteria help us in digesting the food. By consuming sweeteners, we may upset the balance, which can lead us to develop indigestion and other issues to worry about.

Stress and Sugar

It is of no surprise that those who suffer from chronic stress often find it soothing to consume sweet and sugary items. This is their way to reduce stress and calm their nerves. However, as we continue to consume more sugar, thinking that it will help us remain calm, we are also building up a tolerance. Soon, one may need to consume a lot more sugar or go the opposite and avoid it, but both are scenarios which can have negative effects. The former will push the person into being hyperactive and experiencing high-sugar levels and the symptoms that brings. The latter will push a person to stress even more than usual as they will not be able to get their "fix" for the day.

The Obvious Bias

After going through this extensive and slightly intimidating chapter, one thing is certain; everything we are told about sugar is biased. We are constantly fed with biased statements or partial information, all of which goes on to create a sense of want and desire. The only people to benefit from this situation are the ones who create and sell these products. We, the consumers, are far from that.

To give you an idea of how much sugar is being consumed, here are some cold and hard facts to digest.

- Around the time when the United States of America was founded as a country, American citizens consumed around four pounds of sugar every year. That number spiked to 20 pounds every year just a century later. In the mid-1990s, the average American citizen was consuming 120 pounds of sugar every single year. Alarming right? Wait till you learn how much we are consuming today.
- Today, it is estimated that the average American consumes around 160 pounds of sugar every year. That is a massive leap. From 20 pounds to a mind-boggling 160 pounds is a dramatic increase. It does seem a lot,

doesn't it? It breaks down to around 16 ounces of sweetened beverage every day.

Of course, the culprits here continue to blast away the idea that sugar is bad, claiming that they use "latest and cutting-edge technologies that make our products super safe to consume," but that is nothing more than a sales pitch. All they are interested in is keeping their bank account reeling in money from the ill-informed souls who place their trust in them.

All in all, things aren't looking bright for us. It is very hard to try and avoid sugar that harms us. Hard, but not impossible, and for now, that is all the room we need to get started.

Remember this—if it isn't natural, it isn't going in the house. Stick to that, and you start changing things for yourself. The results may not be immediate, but I assure you, you will be thanking yourself later for doing this today.

Well, that was a significantly long chemistry lesson, wasn't it? It is time for me to put aside my chemistry classes, and for us to start looking at something a little more interesting. From here on out, everything that I will teach you will make sense, because now you know all the science.

A SUGAR-FREE DIET FOR YOU

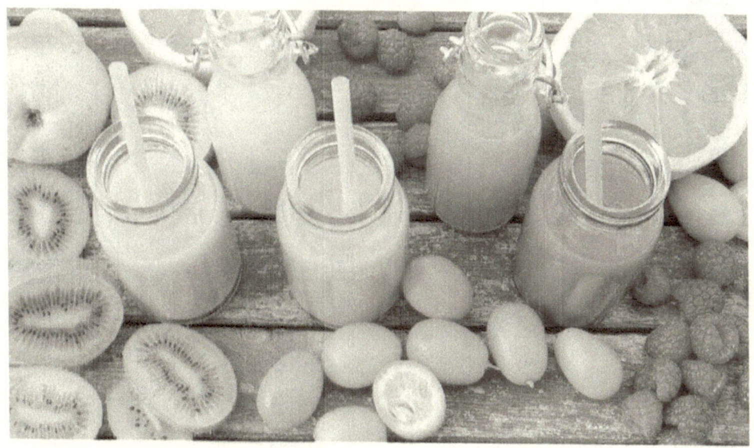

In this chapter, we will fully discover just why we need this kind of diet. We will also get to debunk some myths surrounding the entire idea of sugar-free diets. It is best that you come to know these as they can often be misleading and result in you making the wrong choices.

We will also be diving into how sugar consumption affects our health in general, and to ensure a neutral approach, the pros and cons of the sugar-free diet. Everything has its pros and cons, which is why it is best to learn these as you go along. These will help you in making an informed decision about the type of diet you intend to follow for a healthier lifestyle.

STEPPING INTO THE SUGAR-FREE ZONE

The first thing to notice here is that as soon as we shift to a sugar-free diet, things change. For starters, we cut down on virtually all kinds of sugar intake. We cut down sugar excess completely, but that does not mean that you are consuming zero sugar.

It is absolutely imperative that you understand that there is always a trace of sugar that remains, and depending on the type of food you eat, it may just be negligible in quantity. With such a small trace of sugar, you are not at risk of being harmed by it at all.

Almost everything we consume has glucose, and we saw that in the previous chapter in detail. This means that even though we will adopt a sugar-free diet, there is some trace of it that remains, and this is important to keep in mind as we move forward.

The 21-day sugar-free diet that I have planned for you will of course be both sugar and carb free. However, bear in mind that carbs are a very complex form of sugar, meaning that hints of them may still remain. The diet plan we will learn will not exclude fiber.

Knowing How Much is Enough

The best way to get started is to learn directly from the source. Since we are talking about recommended sugar intake per day, which ultimately falls under the canopy of health, nothing holds more authority than the World Health Organization (WHO).

According to their 2015 published guidelines, it has been recommended that we limit our consumption of added sugar to 5% of our total calories every day. This means that you should limit your added sugar intake to around 25 grams. To give you an idea of how much that is, an average teaspoon of sugar is around four grams in weight.

Nutritionists have gone on to suggest that a healthy American average adult should only get around 10% of their calories from sugar. Bear in mind this is plain sugar we are talking about, not the added sugar forms. If we do the math here, it comes to roughly around 13.3 teaspoons of sugar, based on 2,000 calories per day. The alarming fact, however, is that the current average is above that, and I mean really above that. We currently consume around 42.5 teaspoons per day, and that is a beyond excessive amount (New Hampshire Department of Health and Human Services, n.d.).

By limiting ourselves to under 10%, we are minimizing the risks of developing unhealthy habits and steering ourselves clear of unwanted and problematic health issues, such as obesity. It also minimizes the risk of dental caries.

In the previous chapter, we learned that we are currently consuming around 160 pounds, or 72.5 kilograms of sugar every year. How does that fare then? Let us do some basic mathematics to analyze if we are doing any good.

If we follow the above rule of 10%, it means that we should consume a maximum of 50 grams, give or take, every day. If we were to multiply that number with the number of days in a year, or 365, we end up with 18,250 grams a year. That is in grams, and to convert that into kilograms, we simply divide the figure by 1,000, as there are 1,000 grams that make up a kilo. The results are, well, shocking, to put it mildly.

$$18,250 / 1000 = 18.25 \ Kilograms$$

The above is how much we should be consuming at most. The current average, however, is so far off, it literally is poles apart. There is an alarming difference of 54.25 kilograms, and all of that is excess sugar that we continue to consume today. This means, we are taking 198.6 grams of sugar a day, almost four times as high as the recommended limit. That is more than enough to invite havoc and chaos in our lives. Obesity is not even the worst of the problems as such an excess amount will rot us from within and leave us in a world full of miseries.

This goes to shed light on just why so many people in the world continue to suffer from various health issues, and ultimately death, related to excessive consumption of sugar. This is the harsh reality that exists. The big companies can try all they like to sugar coat this fact, distort it, and claim that things are improving, but the fact remains that sugar is wreaking havoc on the Earth.

Whether you are overweight or otherwise, a high sugar intake spells trouble, period. There is often the factor of "So what?" that tends to jump out of nowhere. I have seen many who tell me to trust them because "just a little never hurt anybody," and a few months later, I have seen them worried sick about their extra pounds. By following a sugar-free diet, we skip the horrible aspects and jump straight into the world of benefits.

It does not matter if you are overweight or not, a sugar-free diet is not limited to a specific group of people. Anyone who intends to lead a healthy and enjoyable life can take part in the sugar-free movement and start on this incredible diet. The results are far more than just fascinating, and they will go on to provide benefit after benefit for the rest of your life.

We will certainly talk in detail about how a sugar-free diet helps. For now, though, we will first learn some of the most commonly reported issues high sugar consumption can bring our way. By being aware, we will have a clearer idea why it is necessary to make the change at this point in time and steer clear of these issues which are almost inevitable for anyone who pushes their luck with sugar.

Obesity

I have mentioned obesity quite a few times, so this one may no longer be of surprise to anyone by now. However, regardless of how many times I go on to refer to obesity, the problem is still a significant one.

Obesity isn't just about gaining excess weight; it is a condition that invites other ailments to come our way. Obesity is a problem that is not limited to the United States alone. People all over the world are suffering from this dreadful condition, and it is also unfortunate to know that many have even died owing to obesity. This makes it all the more important to understand how sugar goes on to be the main culprit behind obesity.

Sodas and fruit juices (which are processed or treated with chemicals and preservatives) contain high volumes of fructose. When we go on to consume fructose, it naturally increases our hunger, more than glucose does. Since we feel hungrier, we continue to consume more food. There comes a point where we start consuming excess amounts of fructose, and that is where a hormone responsible to tell our body to stop eating, called leptin, starts facing resistance. Since our body does not know how to stop in time any longer, we end up consuming more sugar than it can actually handle.

This excessive intake is what starts making room for weight gain. What's more, if we continue consuming these sugary drinks, we also risk an increased amount of something called visceral fat within our bodies. This is a deep belly fat which is generally associated with diabetes and numerous heart diseases (Kubala, 2018). Furthermore, there are a number of research studies that go on to show that people who consume sugary drinks and beverages gain more weight than those who don't.

Diabetes

Whenever we mention obesity, diabetes is bound to make an appearance, which has more to do with the fact that obesity is a leading cause of diabetes. In the last 30 years or so, the existence of diabetes has more than doubled, making it one of the most common ailments people suffer from today (Kubala, 2018).

Apart from obesity, another major link that has been confirmed by researchers worldwide is between excessive sugar consumption and diabetes. Now, imagine a person who consumes excessive sugar and is obese as well. In such a case, it's only a matter of time before diabetes makes its grand entrance.

Prolonged high-sugar consumption is known to cause resistance to naturally formed insulin, which is a hormone whose job is to regulate blood sugar levels. It is secreted by the pancreas, and if it faces resistance, the pancreas stops producing insulin at normal rates. This is why those suffering from diabetes often require additional insulin to help regulate the blood sugar within the body.

When insulin is restricted, blood sugar levels rise dramatically, and the higher they go, the riskier it gets for a person. A healthy person, who may not have diabetes, will soon be struggling to avoid it. They may either end up with type one or type two diabetes.

According to a population study that comprised over 175 countries worldwide, it was found that the risk of developing this dreadful ailment grew by 1.1% every time one consumes 150 g of sugar. This is roughly equivalent to one can of regular soda drink (Basu et al., 2013).

If you think that is bad enough, here is yet another finding that leaves many startled. Anyone who consumes fruit juices or any other sweetened beverage is more likely to end up developing diabetes.

All in all, obesity and the insulin resistance that these sugary drinks cause are classic symptoms of developing type two diabetes, and that is the worst type of diabetes a person can have.

Metabolic Syndrome (formerly Syndrome X)

Prolonged consumption of high or excessive sugar can also lead to something called Metabolic Syndrome. This is a cluster of risk factors, including but not limited to:

- high blood pressure
- high triglycerides
- high blood sugar
- low HDL cholesterol
- belly fat

All of these, combined, increase the risk of developing type two diabetes and other heart conditions. What's more, this is as common as pimples or the common cold, and that means almost every other person is prone to developing this issue.

The American Heart Association reports that 47 million Americans are currently suffering from metabolic syndrome, and that equates to one out of every six people. To make matters worse, its symptoms aren't exactly "well defined" either as there is plenty about it that still evades the eyes of researchers (Web MD, n.d.).

The good news is that this syndrome can be brought under control, but it will require you to adopt a lifelong change of diet and habits, including exercise, physical activities, and a sugar-free diet.

A leading cause of developing the mysterious syndrome X is thought to be insulin resistance. Other possible causes are identified as:

- obesity
- unhealthy lifestyle
- smoking
- hormonal imbalance

All of the above causes are far too common, which is why there is a staggering number of people suffering from this condition. It is not exactly an ailment in itself, but a group of risk factors which can then go on to cause major problems.

Other Conditions and Ailments

Apart from the three we discussed above, there are many other issues which a person can develop should they continue to consume excessive sugar on a regular basis. None of these is pleasant, and almost each can prove to be fatal, if left unchecked or unattended. Let us look at each one of these briefly, just so we can have a clearer picture of just how much damage excessive sugar can cause.

1. Increased risk of heart disease
2. Acne problems
3. Possibly increase in risk of cancer
4. Increased risk of depression
5. Acceleration of the skin aging process
6. Increase in cellular aging
7. Lack of Energy
8. Fatty liver

So far, it is evident that sugar is doing more harm to us than we originally thought. We are being exposed to acne problems, heart issues, fluctuating blood pressure, and so much more. All of which goes on to show that sugar is something we should all learn to avoid at all costs. High-sugar consumption brings with itself an inevitable future, one that no one wishes to face or experience.

BUSTING THE MYTHS

To make things easier, I will list each myth and discuss briefly what it involves, and if there is any truth to it.

Every sugar is bad

Right away, we have the biggest myth that stands in our way. According to this one, every type of sugar that exists is bad. If you have been following the book closely so far, you will already know where this myth stands, and if there is any truth in it.

Experts continue to emphasize that we should all be consuming less sugar. What people fail to realize is that they are referring to the added sugar, not sugar itself. There is a difference between the two, as we have already seen in the previous chapters.

Natural sugar comes in many forms, and usually with other supporting nutrients, such as fiber or vitamins. These go on to help and reduce the negative impacts of sugar to a negligible level. Added sugar, on the other hand, does not do that. It goes on to cause harm, and it does not come with anything that could soften the blow.

To summarize, fruits, vegetables, and all other natural food items with natural sugar are good to go. The rest must stay out of our diet.

Natural sugars or minimally processed sugars are a better choice

Well, there is something that must be admitted. Minimally processed sugars do have an edge over the processed ones. They come with higher quantities of nutrients compared to their processed counterparts, but even that higher count is fractional, and that is not enough to cause any measurable impact on our health.

All of these, minimal or otherwise, still go on to have the same results and impact on your overall weight.

Sugar must be cut out from life for good

Okay, I honestly do struggle with this one. If we cut out sugar completely, we end up not receiving the required energy we need to allow our brain and other parts of the body to function. Right away, there is a major flaw with this myth.

Moreover, there are many health organizations that have agreed to the fact that there is some room for sugar in our healthy diets. Previously, we have come across the fact that

WHO and other institutions have gone on to say that we should limit sugar to around 10% at most. They never said anything about eliminating it completely.

There is no way you can avoid sugar

True. There is no possible way that you can go on to avoid sugar. However, that does not mean that you cannot control the amount of sugar you consume.

It is reported that 75% of American citizens consume more sugar than the amount mentioned by the World Health Organization (Taylor, 2020). If you aren't too sure of the sugar quantity you consume, you can always rely on your smartphone to log the food you eat. There are many apps available which provide you with a good understanding of what you consume, how much you should consume, and whether you ate as much as you should have. Using such apps should give you a fair idea of how much sugar you are consuming. You can then go on to start and limit your intake by either removing or replacing some food item with another which has less sugar.

Sugar makes you sick

If being sick here means having nausea, then this myth is completely irrelevant. However, that is not what this myth is about. The fact is that eating high quantities of sugar can shave off quite a few years from your life as the excess amount will lead you into developing some or a lot of the ailments and diseases we discussed earlier. In this case, the myth stands correct.

As long as you can control your intake of sugar, you should do just fine.

Sugar is addictive

We already know the answer to that, don't we? We discussed something called sugar addiction. However, it is still under debate on whether this condition is real and if sugar addiction is similar to cocaine addiction.

We can either wait for the research to be completed and risk consuming all that sugar, hoping the results will say it isn't a real thing, or we can start limiting it today and be less bothered about the eventual results. I would choose the latter.

Sugar-free replacements are the way to go

Another one that is somewhat answered in our previous chapter. However, in the interest of learning, let us see what's what.

The myth goes that switching from sugar, used to create donuts or as sweeteners for drinks, to sugar-free alternatives is a better move. Weirdly, this swap, if you decide to go for it, could very well backfire and is least likely to have any positive effects on our health.

Aspartame, saccharin, sucralose are the top three names you will come across when searching for sugar-free alternatives.

Unfortunately, these are also linked to weight gain problems. If that wasn't enough, they are also linked to higher risks of developing type two diabetes, syndrome X, and stroke. It is evident where this myth stands after reading all that, right?

You can lose weight by switching to a low- or no-sugar diet

While this may actually sound realistic, there are other factors to consider. Switching to a low-sugar or no-sugar diet does help in reducing weight, but there is another culprit that must also be taken into account—calorie intake.

If you switch to a diet where you do not consume any sugar at all and still consume a significant number of calories, you will still find your weight tipping over the red line. In order to fully take advantage of the low- or no-sugar diet, you will also need to reduce your calorie intake.

Too much sugar makes your kid hyperactive

I will cut to the chase here; there is no such thing as a sugar high. This myth was actually studied by various researchers, and all of them ended with the same conclusion; there is no connection between sugar and kids being hyperactive. It does affect adults, but that is only momentary and that energy boost soon drains away.

Sugar causes cavities

While sugar does have some role to play in messing up your teeth, cavities are actually caused by acid, not sugar. This acid is generally found in beverages, fizzy drinks, or other sources of acid found in various food items.

Sugar causes all health problems

Sugar causes some, not all. Earlier in the book, we learned how much damage sugar does. However, the rest is caused by a million other variables. Blaming sugar alone would neither be right nor logical.

These were some of the myths which were essential for you to know. Had you not known these, you may have gone on to add or take away something from your life unnecessarily.

BENEFITS OF CUTTING OUT SUGAR

Now that the myths have been discussed, let us quickly look at some of the health benefits you can expect once you start to cut down on sugar.

There are many benefits that come to mind once you start to cut down on sugar, but to ensure that we touch base with each one of these, I decided to put together a list, just to make things a lot easier for everyone. I am not implying that everyone will experience the same benefits because there are many other variables to consider such as age, weight, height, any underlying condition, family history of diabetes, etc.

However, for this list, we will put those variables aside and look at some of the most commonly reported benefits of cutting down sugar.

Reduces risk for cardiovascular conditions and obesity

If we adopt a healthier diet option, we immediately take away the biggest risks of them all. By sticking to a no-sugar or a low-sugar diet, we significantly reduce the risk of developing any cardiovascular conditions, and we virtually eradicate the chance of ever having to worry about obesity.

Cuts risk of developing diabetes

Besides being able to lose weight, a healthier diet also allows us to cut down the risk of developing diabetes, especially the dreadful type two diabetes.

Improves skin

Who doesn't want to have radiant skin these days? By switching to a healthier diet, you allow your skin to feel fresh and can be free of any acne problems. Besides, you do not have to worry about aging either as a healthier diet will ensure you never exceed your sugar levels for the day.

Teeth-friendly

Our teeth are a major part of our personality, whether people care to admit it or not. Imagine someone who looks handsome, but the instance this person smiles, he has massively stained, blackish teeth, which will put off every person around him. That is what excessive sugar can do to your teeth.

A healthier diet ensures that your teeth are never exposed to a harmful quantity of sugar. Also, there are many other things which a healthy diet ensures your teeth remain clear of, leaving you with every reason to smile brightly.

Lasting energy at your disposal

Sugar takes away energy, and we have come to a point where we are far too familiar with how that happens. The good news is that we can easily regain the energy levels we would normally have by cutting down on sugar. It is as simple as that.

The switch from a regular diet to a healthier diet allows you to consume complex carbs, healthier fats, and proteins, all of which are a terrific formula to provide you with sustainable energy.

Goodbye abdominal fats

Yet another massive health benefit, and also another one we already read about previously. By not consuming high amounts of sugar, we are certainly ensuring that our bodies start losing weight, and also curbing any risk of developing those stubborn abdominal fats. This means we will not have to worry about a belly that may be bulging out of proportion, and we will be able to fit into our favorite jeans with no worries at all.

All of this only goes to show that sugar is bad, and that adopting a sugar-free or low-sugar diet is the way to go. We have also busted several myths, and even looked at both the benefits and the damages. However, jumping into a sugar-free diet now would be too soon because there are some pros and cons which everyone should be aware of.

THE PROS AND CONS

Straight away, I will get on with the things you can eat and the ones which are a clear no-no.

Things You can Enjoy

- whole grains
- green, leafy vegetables (either raw or cooked)
- fruits (berries and citrus fruits)
- fatty fish
- beans and legumes
- nuts and seeds
- sweet potatoes
- herbs and spices
- lean protein

Things to Avoid

- fruits with high glycemic index scale ratings
- refined sugar
- white bread
- flour
- alcohol (excess)
- packaged snacks (chips or pretzels)
- sugary drinks (Capritto, 2020)

"That's not too bad, is it?" Certainly not. Yes, we may not be able to consume some of our favorite drinks or use flour as often as we normally would, but I assure you, with the recipes I have lined up for your 21-day sugar-free diet, you will never miss these ever again.

Time for us to explore the pros and cons, considering that we intend to go ahead with the sugar-free diet. There are several of these, and they require a person to carefully assess them and see if such a diet can help them with their targets. Of course, in an ideal world, we would all stick to a sugar-free diet, not because of the numerous benefits, but because it is almost certain that we will go on to lead a healthier life.

Pros

A sugar-free diet can:

- help with weight loss
- promote the heart's health
- improve mental health as well
- lower the risk of any diabetes
- always be customized to suit your taste better
- be extremely easy and have plentiful recipes too

Cons

On the opposite end of the scale, a sugar-free diet:

- is not at all helpful for intense workouts
- can at times be complicated
- can rarely trigger eating disorders

While the pros are pretty much self-explanatory, I would like to highlight the cons a little, just to add transparency and give everyone a fair understanding of what they are about to adopt.

For people who love intense workouts, such as body builders, intense weightlifters, marathon participants, and athletes looking forward to the Olympics, this is not the kind of diet for you. Your bodies will need to build all that muscle just to cope up with the extreme exertion required. A sugar-free diet will not allow you to do that. To build muscles, you may be required to rely on additional protein and carbohydrate sources, hence overruling the limits of the sugar-free diet.

A sugar-free diet is in no way easy to manage. It takes time, effort, and quite a bit of understanding before you are able to fully understand how it works. Take your own self, as an example. You are reading through so much detail, just so you can understand the entire science that goes into making a sugar-free diet what it is. You will also need to look out for labels and the information they provide and calculate how many calories you can consume and when you have reached a limit for the day.

It is a cumbersome task, especially for beginners. The change from processed food to cooking entire meals at home requires commitment, and not everyone may have the time or resources to do that. However, rest assured that those who manage to continue doing this for a while will develop a habit, and the rest will just be routine work. The results, however, will be rewarding enough to compensate for all the hard work that you put in.

Sugar-free diets can sometimes pose a risk of developing certain eating disorders. Given the nature of this diet and what it is capable of doing, it is only normal that this type of diet flirts with the border between diet and obsession. Quite often people are caught up in the hype and instead of focusing on the diet itself, they start becoming obsessed, labeling food good or bad on their own.

Of course, all of these are not always the case; however, it is good that you now know what you are about to start. With that said, it is time to move to our next chapter and start uncovering how much sugar exists around us. You might be surprised by what you may find in the next chapter, but once again, the more you know the easier it will be for you to avoid perils that may lie right ahead.

3

BEWARE! SUGAR IS EVERYWHERE

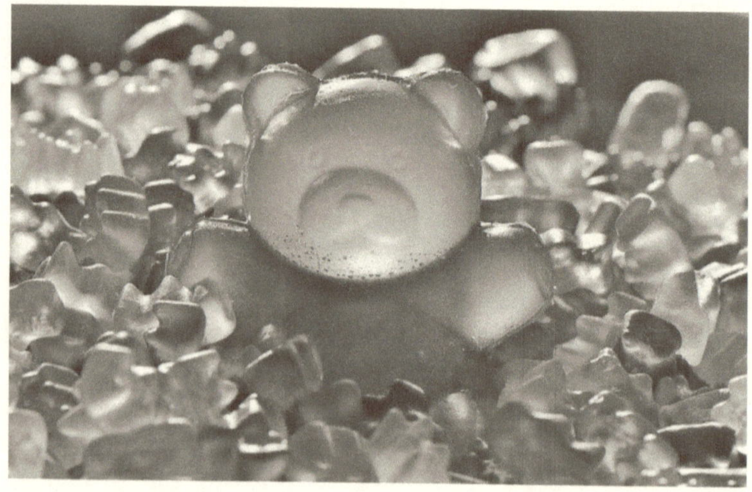

In this chapter, we will explore how some companies we believe to be trustworthy continue to hide away the facts which we should know in the first place. We will also shed light on some of the compliant and noncompliant food as per our diet, as well as learn how to read labels correctly, just so we know if there is any hidden sugar. Finally, we will dive in a little deeper to see if dried fruits, honey, and alcohol are okay to be consumed.

HIDING IN PLAIN SIGHT

One of the biggest ways companies continue to make money is not by selling us lies, but only sharing half of the truth. This is normally some kind of fact that is used as a unique selling point for any product or company to attract more attention. Marketing students may be able to understand what I am on about, but the fact is, you do not need to be a marketing student to figure out that these unique selling points are only showing half of the picture.

Let us be honest, when was the last time you saw a Red Bull can warn that it has a high-sugar content? Probably never. This is why it is important for us to understand how companies and organizations use various methods to hide away so much information from us. I will list down eight of these ways to give everyone a clear understanding of how information is cleverly hidden from us. With careful observation, you can actually find out if a product is holding back on something or not.

Making Sugar Sound Cool

I mentioned how companies go on to invest billions of dollars into research and development, and despite the massive amounts, the only good that comes out of such research benefits them and them alone. Consumers, however, end up with nothing more than some fancy words, which try to make sugar sound safer and cooler.

We are no stranger to these names. In fact, many of us may have already come across such names in a variety of products. Companies go on to hire creative minds to ensure that they can come up with some way to make sugar more acceptable, just so their products continue to sell. The more they sell, the more they earn. What happens to the consumers, well, that is of small concern to them. This means it is up to us to keep an eye out for some of these names which I have come across so far.

Better Ways of Saying Dry Sugar

I understand dry ice, but dry sugar was certainly one that raised my eyebrow. If companies start being honest, they will end up mentioning that their product uses dry sugar as a part of their ingredients, which would effectively serve a massive blow to the product's sales figures. Instead, there are many names which effectively mean the same as dry sugar, but these are accepted because almost no one has an idea of what they are looking at. The information is there, but it is hiding in plain sight, and these companies do little to nothing to notify the consumers of what they are about to consume. Some names that I have seen which are used instead of dry sugar are:

- beet sugar
- barley malt
- buttered sugar
- brown sugar
- cane sugar
- cane juice crystals
- caster sugar
- corn sweetener
- coconut sugar
- crystalline fructose
- dextran or malt powder
- date sugar
- ethyl maltol
- golden sugar
- fruit juice concentrate
- invert sugar
- maltose
- maltodextrin
- muscovado sugar
- palm sugar
- panela
- organic raw sugar
- evaporated cane juice
- rapadura sugar
- confectioner's sugar (powdered)

Quite a list of names, isn't it? I am sure you may have come across a few already. I would also encourage you to write these down in a notebook or a smartphone notes app. The next time you are in the kitchen or the pantry, or even out to do groceries, make sure you check the ingredients and see if you come across any of these. However, that is not the end of the list either. Here are some other things to consider and keep a lookout for.

Syrups

Apart from sugar being added in the form of dry sugar, there are many products where sugar is added in the form of syrups. These syrups are generally thick in nature, and they are made using extremely large quantities of sugar. By dissolving this large quantity of sugar, you end up with what we call a syrup. Of course, this is already raising alarms for us, considering that a teaspoon of syrup alone will knock our sugar intake levels off balance. Imagine how much syrup is used to make various products and how we easily consume them without realizing just how much trouble we are inviting.

Nowadays, the companies which make such products using syrups are well aware of the problems it will cause them if they start to print out the real names. Just like the companies which came up with new and innovative ways to say dry sugar, these companies have also come up with a variety of names they continue to use. Some of these names are:

- agave nectar

- golden syrup
- carob syrup
- honey
- high-fructose corn syrup
- malt syrup
- molasses
- maple syrup
- oat syrup
- rice syrup
- rice bran syrup

Now, you have a complete list of names to keep an eye out for. To make the most of your diet, make sure you refrain from using products with any of these names.

Using a Variety of Sugars

There is a specific format which companies follow when mentioning their ingredients. The main ingredients are always listed first. However, "the more of one item, the higher up on the list it appears" (West, 2019).

Food manufacturers around the world have been known to take advantage of this. They go on to use three or four types of sugar, in smaller quantities, to ensure that the consumers still believe they are consuming less sugar, and the companies continue to make profits.

When companies use three to four different sugars, they appear further down the list, giving an impression that the product contains low sugar levels, whereas it still remains as the main ingredient.

To give you a real-life example, there is a certain protein bar, portrayed as being one of the healthiest in the market, that contains around 7.5 teaspoons or 30 grams of sugar in just a single bar.

The good news is that you already know the most common names used to hide away the fact that sugar is used in products. Use these names and find out which products have multiple layers of sugar mentioned. It will make it a lot easier to avoid high-sugar consumption, and you will easily be able to steer clear of the horrible issues that sugar brings.

Sugar in Products You Least Expect

Okay, there is no rocket science involved in guessing that food items, such as cakes and cookies, are brimming with sugar content. However, it might be a bit confusing and a little surprising to some that food companies continue to add sugar in products where it is least expected. These products may not even be sweet to begin with. Some fine examples are spaghetti sauce, breakfast cereals, and yogurt.

To further highlight what I am talking about, some yogurts within the market may contain as much as six teaspoons of sugar. That is around 29 grams of sugar, and that is quite a shocking amount, considering that yogurt is not even considered to be a sweet product.

The big takeaway is to ensure that you check the label before you make your purchase. The product may be portrayed as healthy, but it is always a good idea to check the label, just to be sure.

Using Healthy Sugar, Not Sucrose

We know what sucrose is. However, people do not realize how easily these giant companies continue to claim that they are using "healthier" alternatives, but the truth is far from it.

These companies continue to use unrefined sweeteners, which are normally made using fruits, flowers, saps, or some kind of plant seeds. I mentioned agave nectar in the previous list, and that is a prime example of what I am talking about.

You will often find labels claiming "contains no refined sugar" or something in the lines of "refined sugar-free," and the only thing they mean is that they don't contain white sugar. They are never free of sugar completely.

I do admit that these sugars have a lower glycemic index (GI) score; however, you do not get many nutrients, and any unrefined sugar is, whether we like it or not, added sugar.

If you are consuming more sugar, it does not matter if you swap your sugar of choice to one that holds a lesser GI score. Furthermore, there is no specific evidence to suggest that a person would benefit from such a swap.

Below are some of the most common high-sugar sweeteners which many go on a label as healthier alternatives:

- agave syrup
- coconut sugar
- birch syrup
- honey
- raw sugar
- maple syrup
- sugar beet syrup
- cane sugar

Combination of Added Sugars and Natural Sugars

When we consume fruits, vegetables, or dairy products, we may consume more sugar than we need, but that may be okay because we will also be consuming other nutrients such as protein or fiber, which will ensure that our blood sugar levels do not spike. This never happens if we go on to consume added sugar.

Companies continue to use labels which never distinguish between natural sugars and added sugars. What they do instead is to list all types of sugar in a single amount. This further causes confusion, and that leaves us with little to no room for fully understanding how much natural sugar or added sugar is present within a food item.

The best way to get about this is to ensure that you stick to unprocessed, whole food items. Try and avoid any processed and packaged food items, and you will ensure that the only sugar that you consume is the one that forms naturally.

Sprinkling Health Claims

You may come across labels or packages which say the product is "Natural" or "Healthy," and this should give you an indication that there is something the manufacturers are not ready to confess.

Other labels to keep an eye out for include:

- low fat
- diet
- light

Smaller Portion Sizes

Companies often use a strategy through which they distort our understanding of the product. They do so by deliberately listing a smaller portion size, and that naturally leads to a lower sugar consumption count. People are often too quick to skim through the sugar value, without paying attention to the fact that the portion size may be smaller than the one we normally consume.

When people overlook this, they continue to eat normal portion sizes, thinking that they are consuming less sugar.

Another example to see is that of a mini-pizza or a bottle of soda. These generally contain several servings. However, the reality is that we consume more than the serving size mentioned on the label. Sometimes, these serving sizes are ridiculously small, making it very easy to spot that the company is trying their best to avoid giving out the real value of sugar a person might consume in a regular serving size.

A good idea is to ensure that you always pay attention to the serving size these products reflect. Generally, small food items have more than a single serving, and these are the ones that we end up consuming more than we need.

Low Sugar with a Sweeter Twist

There are a lot of famous low-sugar product lineups these days within the market. While they continue to sell nicely, some-times, the people who make these come up with more sweet-ened versions of these products. This means that they will pack in more sugary content within their products, just to give them the sweeter taste.

A typical example of the above is that of breakfast cereals. A whole-grain cereal of your choice, which would normally be low in sugar, will then go on to be released with a new pack-aging and so-called "added flavors" to give them that enhanced taste. Quite a lot of people fall for this trap, thinking that this new type of flavor is still as healthy as the original product, and that is far from the reality.

The "Yes" and the "No"

In the previous chapter, we briefly touched upon the type of food you can go on to eat, and those which you should avoid. These are called compliant and noncompliant food items.

Compliant food items are generally the ones containing natural or healthier sugar contents. These are free of any added sugar, and they do not generally pose any risk to health. Noncompliant food items are the ones which are neither recommended nor required by those who follow a sugar-free diet lifestyle. These have added sugar content and can often prove to be problematic in nature.

Below is a list of food items, starting from the one that is loaded with extra sugar, all the way to food items with the least or virtually no sugar at all. If you wish to get going on a lower sugar content lifestyle, it is a good idea to consult this list and start cutting down or minimizing the use of the sugar heavy items in your daily intake. This will serve as your next step in getting a head start on a sugar-free diet.

1. **Food with added sugar** – Candies, sweetened drinks, pastries, sweetened foods and many more
2. **Refined grains** – White bread, pasta, white rice, bagels, crackers, baked goods; these are some of the items which fall into this category.
3. **Whole grains or starches** – These include brown rice, whole-grain bread, quinoa, and oats.
4. **Fruits** – Bananas, apples, pineapples, peaches, berries, pears, and many others.
5. **Starchy vegetables** – Potatoes, carrots, squash, pumpkins, beets, and so on.
6. **Green vegetables** – Broccoli, asparagus, cabbage, spinach, lettuce, brussels sprouts, and some others.

Eliminating the top one and cutting down on the rest may seem like an ideal move, but you do not have to push yourself to the brink of starvation at all. Just removing the first two categories alone will have significant results. However, as we move ahead and discover the recipes, we will learn what kind of food items are best to be used every day.

Another good way to go would be to identify the group where most of the food you eat currently belongs and replace it with the one underneath it. You can add more items to your general diet, and that also should provide you with a healthier outcome. For example, if you are someone who consumes a lot of pastries, consider swapping that with fruits.

Fats – Do we need them?

Fats are nutrients, just like proteins and carbohydrates, and this means that our bodies rely on these. Our body gets energy from fats, and these go on to help absorb vitamins. This may also seem a bit surprising, but fats protect our heart and our brain and ensure that they remain healthy. Take away the fats from our bodies, and we end up risking everything. If you don't provide your body what it needs, you could end up doing harm to your health.

The biggest misconception about fats is that they cause you to gain weight, meaning we can no longer fit into the jeans of our choice, and so on. The reality is that there are good fats and then there are bad fats, and both of them are poles apart.

The good fats, such as omega-3s, go on to brighten our moods, give us all the mental energy we need to go through the day, and allow us to control our weight better. The bad fats, on the other hand, aim to throw our bodies off balance. These are the ones we should watch out for as they can easily add weight, cause harm to our internal organs, and do a lot more damage.

It is important for us to know just why we need good fats and how these can go on to help us maintain better weight and be in better shape.

Understanding Cholesterol

We begin with dietary fat. It plays an important role in influencing our cholesterol levels. While many believe that cholesterol is bad, it is not the case. Our body actually needs cholesterol to function properly. It is a wax-like, fatty substance that flows around our body. However, the levels of cholesterol can be influenced by the kind of diet we eat. If we are not careful and if we continue to consume bad fats, our cholesterol levels can spike up, leading to clogged arteries, and we all know what that leads to.

When it comes to dietary fats, there are both good and bad types of cholesterols.

- LDL cholesterol is the one to watch out for. It is also referred to as the bad cholesterol.
- HDL cholesterol is the polar opposite of LDL cholesterol. This means that this is the good cholesterol, and that it is present naturally within our blood.
- The objective should always be to ensure that HDL cholesterol remains high while LDL cholesterol remains low, to ensure we avoid any heart diseases or stroke.

This means that we must aim to consume good fats as these go on to boost our HDL cholesterol count while lowering the LDL cholesterol. However, to do that, let us first understand both the good and the bad fats.

The Good vs. The Bad

Both monounsaturated and polyunsaturated fats are known as good fats. They are good for the heart and cholesterol and have great overall health benefits. Using these fats will allow you to:

- lower bad LDL cholesterol levels
- increase HDL cholesterol levels
- lower risk of developing heart diseases or stroke
- prevent irregular or abnormal heart rhythms
- lower blood pressure
- lower triglycerides which are associated with heart diseases
- fight inflammation
- prevent atherosclerosis

It also should be noted that using these good fats in your diet will allow you to feel satisfied, while ensuring weight loss at the same time. Some good sources for these are:

Monounsaturated Fats

- avocados
- peanut butter
- olive oil, canola oil, peanut oil, and sesame oil
- olives

- nuts (almonds, macadamia, hazelnuts, peanuts, pecans, cashews)

Polyunsaturated Fats

- flaxseeds
- walnuts
- sunflower seeds
- pumpkin seeds
- sesame seeds
- soymilk
- tofu
- fatty fish (such as tuna, salmon, mackerel, trout, herring, sardines)
- fish oil
- soybeans oil
- safflower oil

When it comes to the bad fats, two names generally appear at the top of this list—trans fats and saturated fats. While the naturally occurring trans fat found in meat poses no health risk, it is the artificial versions that we should always avoid. These are considered as the worst type of fats. They can easily spike LDL cholesterol levels while lowering HDL cholesterols significantly. They also cause inflammation, which is directly linked to heart disease, strokes, and other severe conditions. Evidence suggests that these fats also cause insulin resistance, which ultimately leads to type two diabetes.

On the other hand, saturated fats are not as dangerous as trans fats, but they still pose health risks as they too can raise LDL cholesterol levels and cause other problems.

The primary sources for both of these are:

Trans Fats

- packaged snack foods (microwave popcorns, chips, crackers)
- commercially baked pastries, doughnuts, muffins, cookies, pizza dough
- stick margarine
- fried food
- anything that contains hydrogenated or partially hydrogenated vegetable oil (Segal, 2019)

Saturated Fats

- butter
- ice cream
- red meat (lamb, beef, pork)
- chicken skin
- lard
- whole-fat dairy products
- tropical oils

Steer clear of these or at least limit them as much as you can. If your body is bombarded by unhealthy and bad fats, you will experience more problems than your body might be able to handle. The good fats, on the other hand, are extremely good and provide our body with sufficient benefits, thus ensuring that our body remains fit and energized, without facing any of the risks associated with the bad fats.

Fiber

Just like the good fats, our bodies also need fiber. It is because of fiber that we are able to consume natural sugars, without worrying about it pushing our blood sugar levels through the roof. It is also a beneficial nutrient as it helps in the digestion process and allows us to feel full and satisfied after a meal. Fiber is known to reduce absorption of fructose in our digestive system, hence limiting or keeping our blood sugar levels under control.

Besides, fiber is also known to help maintain a healthy weight while lowering the risk of diabetes. It also reduces the risk of developing heart conditions and certain types of cancer.

Fiber also helps in normalizing bowel movements. This means that it helps those who may be suffering from constipation. It is also helpful if you suffer from loose, watery stools as fiber absorbs water and solidifies the stool to allow easier passage.

Apart from helping with bowel movement, fiber also lowers bad cholesterol levels. Previously, we learned about LDL cholesterol levels, and fiber is yet another way to ensure these are kept under check.

Furthermore, fiber also helps in regulating blood sugar levels. This is why people who may be suffering from diabetes are often recommended to add fiber into their diets.

Some good sources for fiber include:

- fruits
- vegetables
- whole-grain products
- nuts and seeds
- beans, peas and many other legumes (Mayo Clinic, 2018)

Low GI is Good

GI stands for Glycemic Index. This is a ranking of carbohydrates on a scale of zero to 100. This ranking is used to determine how each of these carbohydrates raises blood sugar levels after they are consumed. Carbohydrates which go on to cause blood sugar levels to fluctuate higher are given a higher number. The ones with a lower ranking are generally the best ones to target as they do not cause blood sugar levels to fluctuate as rapidly and are absorbed slowly. They are also considered as the secret to a long and healthy life.

Generally speaking, a low GI food would have a ranking from zero to 55. Food items with a medium GI score would stand between 56 to 69. Anything above 69 is considered as a food item with a high GI score (Villines, 2019).

The Glycemic Index Foundation goes on to recommend an average dietary GI score of 45 as providing the best health benefits. With that said, there are a few things to bear in mind. GI values can fluctuate, depending on how the food item is being consumed.

If you are cooking a food item, the GI score tends to rise. A pasta, for example, will have a lower GI score initially as compared to the same pasta when cooked and softened. Similarly, food processing also goes on to raise GI scores. Surprisingly, fruits which are ripe have higher GI scores than their younger counterparts. Finally, the type of food we eat along with the food source affects the GI value as well. Fiber is known to reduce the GI score, so if you were to consume fiber with another food item, it would automatically lower the overall GI value.

Some good examples of lower GI food items include:

- barley
- nonstarchy vegetables
- whole grain pasta
- legumes
- bulgur

- whole grains
- lentils
- oat bran
- many beans
- steel-cut oatmeal
- brown or wild rice
- muesli
- most of the fruits

Foods with higher GI values include:

- popcorn
- puffed rice
- heavily processed grain
- instant oatmeal
- saltine crackers
- pumpkin
- starchy vegetables
- pretzels
- melons
- corn flakes
- bran flakes
- pineapple

Things You Should Know

Soon, we will be starting with the recipes, but there are a few things you should write down and bear in mind:

1. You will need to avoid fruits for the first 15 days of the diet plan. This is to ensure that you get the help you need for your cravings. It is very easy to be tempted to consume something sweet, just to end the craving. By restricting yourself for the first 15 days, you will have already cut down massively on your sugar intake.
2. There will be some snack and dessert recipes within this book, and they will include the use of fruits. Once again, you will need to avoid those for the first two weeks. After that, it is completely your call.

Reading Labels

Reading labels can be tricky, especially for someone who may have never read a label before or has no idea on how to read them. Fortunately, I do, and I am going to provide you with a step-by-step guide to ensure you learn how to read the labels the next time you do your grocery shopping.

1. Total Sugars – This part of the label generally includes all the sugars, natural or added, present within the product for each serving. There is never a daily value mentioned for this as experts are yet to provide a specific figure. If you are on a low-sugar diet, pay attention to this part of the label.
2. Added Sugars – This is exactly what it sounds like. This part of the label includes all the added sugars, regardless of the fancy names they may have. The daily

value for this is 50 grams, based on a 2,000-calorie daily diet. If you are on a different calorie-per-day diet, this figure will fluctuate accordingly.

The added sugars are generally listed under the total sugars. At times, they reflect how much added sugar is present within the product, while other times they only mention the percentage of daily value (DV).

If the DV is 5% or lower, it is considered to be a low-sugar source. If the DV is 20% or more, it is considered to be a high-sugar source. The next time you are looking at labels, ensure that you pay close attention to these two items.

Reading the label is fairly easy, but without proper guidance, it may often be confusing as a lot of information is present, which can easily baffle a beginner.

Can I consume dried fruits then?

Fruits, when ripe, have a higher GI score. It also means that they will have significant sugar within them, albeit natural. If we were to dry the fruit, would it lower the sugar count?

This may surprise you a little, but dried fruits actually have a higher sugar content than their fresh counterparts. That is because when the fruits are dried, they have shrunk and their volume decreases significantly. If we go on to eat them in larger quantities, we end up consuming excessive sugar quantities. Prolonged use of dried fruits, in significant quantities, can easily pave way for diabetes and other issues.

What about honey? Is that safe?

We all love honey, and there is no denying that. However, just because we love honey does not mean that it is not exactly sugar free. While honey is the sweetest gift of nature, it is to be noted that honey is still counted as added sugar. This means that anything that you may make using honey or even consuming a spoon full of it, would give you the same results.

With that said, it does not mean that you should give up on honey completely and stop enjoying it. WHO recommended that we limit our added sugar intake to 10%, and if you follow those guidelines strictly, you may just be able to enjoy a bit of honey with your meals or breakfast every day.

If you wish to buy honey, ensure that you go for the all-natural honey which you can find at most farms. Aim for raw honey with pollen in it. This lets you know that the honey was not heated or processed.

Remember: Raw honey should not be consumed by infants, pregnant women, babies, or those who may be immune compromised as it is not processed and is unpasteurized.

The best way to use honey is as a replacement for white sugar. White sugar does more harm, and using honey as a replacement will ensure that this harm is limited, and that the blood sugar does not fluctuate as much.

Finally, what about alcohol?

Ah, the one drink that everyone's been thinking about. Just as alcohol can cause us to get into a confused state, it also puts our body in a similar state as well.

Alcohol prevents our liver from producing glucose. This means that the blood sugar levels within our body will either shoot up or fall down. It also should be noted that hypoglycemia can also occur after the night of consuming alcohol.

Since alcohol has a weird effect on the body, people who drink and have diabetes are often recommended to eat something else, to compensate for the expected blood sugar level drops.

Before going out for a drink or two, it is a good idea to check your blood sugar levels. This will allow you to know whether you would need to eat something else or if you will be just fine.

All in all, as long as you are careful of what you consume and how much you end up drinking, the results should be safe enough, and you should be able to enjoy a pleasant evening. If you tend to overdose on these, not only will you wake up with a pounding headache, but you will also have gone fairly above your sugar intake limits for the day. You will then need to put in extra days, just to compensate for what you might have done the other night.

Finally, the time has come to end this chapter and start moving towards the practical aspects of the book. The next chapter will take you through some of the challenges a person may face when they finally decide "I am ready to do this." Pay close attention to the next chapter, take notes, and ensure that you clarify all your doubts, if you have any, because as soon as we are done with the next chapter, the second part of the book starts, and that is where we start cooking.

4

AROUND THE NO-SUGAR DIET - HOW TO HELP YOUR BODY ADJUST TO CHANGE

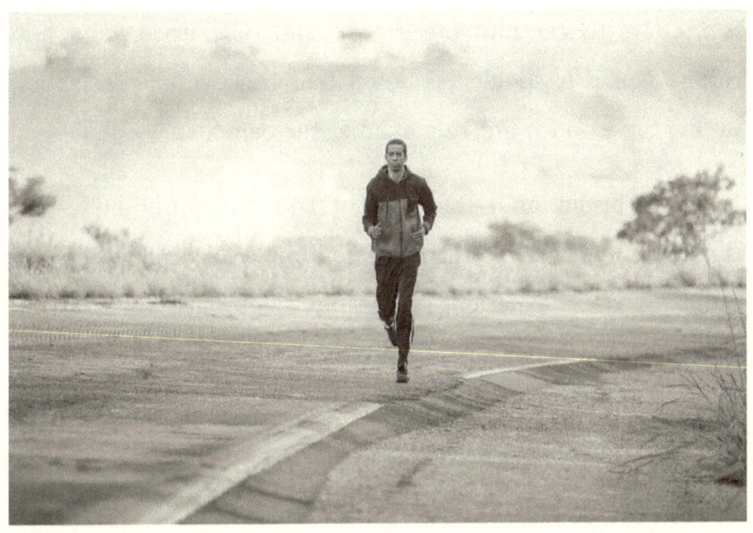

This chapter dives into the kind of challenges and possible effects that you may encounter when undergoing a three-week-long diet. You need to know of these effects so that you are not taken by surprise, nor find yourself struggling to overcome obstacles. Some days may be harder than others, and you may even be tempted to cheat a little, but it is up to you to follow your diet accordingly. This chapter will give you the chance to mentally prepare yourself for these challenges. We will also look into what you can do to carry on after the three-week diet, but that is a different chapter, which we will talk about later.

HOW THE DIET AFFECTS YOUR BODY

The diet that we are about to start stretches on for 21 days. That is 21 days to get into the groove and fully understand how things work. It should be noted that the overall diet should ideally carry on for life, to maximize the benefits.

It would be an understatement if I said that our body goes through some changes during these three weeks. The fact is that our body starts experiencing various symptoms, and knowing about them will help us prepare better, starting from the first week of this life-changing switch.

Week One

Right from the start, you will start experiencing a lack of energy throughout the week. You will feel tired and exhausted and may experience fatigue as well. You will experience headaches as you normally would if you decide to cut down on caffeine, nicotine, or alcohol.

You might be tempted to give in and consume something sweet, but do not fall for your cravings. You will need to fight these temptations and remain determined.

Besides the above, you will also experience mental acuity, and some may go on to experience gastrointestinal distress (Magner, 2018).

Speaking strictly from a medical view, it is not clear why people go on to experience these symptoms. However, if it's any consolation, these symptoms are fairly normal, and you should not feel alarmed by any of these. Research has shown that when sugar is taken out of the equation, the body undergoes similar withdrawal symptoms as it would when ditching drugs (Avena et al., 2008).

Remember how sugar pushes the production of dopamine, the feel-good chemical? Now that we are taking sugar away, our dopamine levels will drop as well. This will lead to cravings, and that can at times be tricky to handle. Besides the decrease in dopamine, our body also experiences another unique change.

There are neurotransmitters called acetylcholine, which are responsible for regulating pain perceptions, and we all have them within us. In the first week of our sugar-free diet, these rise in numbers. This is exactly the kind of chemical reaction that is associated with withdrawal symptoms.

If we were to put science aside and talk in a language everyone can understand, this specific phase is not permanent and should soon end. Earlier, I mentioned that most of these symptoms are felt by almost everyone, but I did leave room there for exception. Not everyone experiences these symptoms, and it is not definite that you will experience them as well.

For those who go on to experience these effects, remind yourself that this phase is temporary and that you need to go through this to experience a better life ahead. A week or two of changes is worth enduring because the reward will be lifelong.

There will be times where you may feel like you have had it and that you want to resume your sugar intake. Do not dive back into the world of candies, pastries, or any other sweet items with added sugar. A better approach would be to eat some fruit, just to ease things a bit. However, there are two things you should remember:

1. The fruit should ideally be one with a lower GI score
2. It should only be used as a last resort. Do not keep munching on fruits throughout the day as that may ruin your efforts.

It will be hard, it will be challenging, and it will certainly be a hectic week. Prepare your mind, and expect the worst to come. Only after preparing for the worst, you might find the entire phase easier.

Week Two

What you will be experiencing in the second week prominently is termed as residual cravings. These are the last few days of craving, and this is why your cravings may max out. The withdrawal symptoms, however, will no longer be a thing to worry about. Most of the withdrawal symptoms will have subsided by now. Those which may remain will fade out within a matter of days.

To combat the cravings, you will need to rely on a lot of proteins, fiber, and healthy fats. You can incorporate these three essentials in your meals, and by consuming them, you will gain all the energy you need to fight the residual cravings.

A meal, which may contain all three important nutrients, will last longer, making you feel fuller for long. This will also allow you to overlook any cravings as you will not feel hungry.

Week Three

After two long and arduous weeks, it is time for the final week to commence. This week will be the best of them all. With no withdrawal symptoms to worry about, and even the residual cravings diminishing to virtually negligible levels, it will be smooth sailing.

Of course, if you make it this far, it means that your body has accepted the changes, and that you too may have changed your meals a bit. Some people switch to unsweetened almond milk while others prefer to settle for Greek yogurt. Whatever the case may be, your body will by now be accustomed to the new diet.

This is also the week where you finally start experiencing the fruits of your hard work. You will no longer have cravings, and you will start losing weight. Yes, you read that right, your weight will start to drop. For those who thought losing weight was not possible, you can measure your weight now and recheck it after the next three weeks, and you will see the difference yourself.

The reason why you start losing weight is because the excess sugar which was once within your body was stored as fats. When the supply of more sugar stops, the body starts to break these fats down and use that as fuel instead. This is exactly the same principle which is followed by the famous Keto diet, and a lot of other diets use the same concept.

Once you start seeing your weight coming down, it will also serve as a morale booster for you. You will now feel more confident than ever before, knowing that you did something that you had been struggling to do for ages. With the weight coming down, you will know that you can do this and that you can see this through.

A word of warning though—you will find yourself instantly drawn to sweet food items at this point. This means that you will need to ensure that you keep these culprits away from you and your diet. The rest of your no-sugar food items will not pose any problems.

With that said, by the end of the third week, you will have completed your 21-day sugar-free diet, and now, you will have everything you need to continue the momentum.

"Well, it does sound easy that way, but are these the only symptoms I will face?"

Withdrawal Symptoms

Before we look at the list of possible symptoms, it is important to remind everyone that not all people will experience them. It is possible that you may not experience any symptoms at all, which will mean that you have already controlled your sugar intake significantly. If you are that lucky person, the entire 21-day sugar-free diet will be just another Tuesday for you.

Mental Symptoms

- depressed mood
- anxiety
- cognitive problems
- disturbed sleep patterns
- cravings

Apart from these mental symptoms, there are some physical symptoms as well which we must all learn and be aware of. These include:

Physical Symptoms

- headaches
- feeling tired
- light-headedness
- nausea

These are some of the most common symptoms reported so far. However, should you experience any other symptom that is not one of the ones listed above, it may be a good idea to check in with your doctor. Some underlying ailments or diseases can often trigger unnatural symptoms, and those must be attended to right away.

Dealing with Symptoms

One way to deal with most symptoms is to get some fresh air, but that is not exactly the healthiest way to go about it. What we need is a way through where we can minimize the effects of these symptoms while ensuring that we continue to remain healthy at the same time. Fortunately, there are some ways through that allow us to do exactly that.

Be Realistic

Being unrealistic will only put us into a more troubling posi-tion. It is not realistic that you can remove or reduce all the sugar sources at once. We need to reduce these added sugar sources one by one, and that is generally a more successful formula to work with.

Remember, the main point is to reduce sources of added sugar to a point that they are virtually nonexistent. Start with the biggest source, and make your way down the list until you know you are consuming sugar under the recommended limit set by various health institutions.

Protein is Your Friend

Protein comes to our rescue, especially in difficult times like these. By adding protein to every meal that you eat, you allow yourself to feel full for longer durations. When you feel full, you will generally not have the urge to eat more food or consume anything else at all.

Protein will also provide you with some energy boost, a perfect way to compensate for the loss of energy owing to the sugar-free diet.

Increase Fiber Intake

We already know what fiber does and how it helps in managing weight, ensuring smooth bowel movements and helping dissolve sugar. What you may not know is that consuming fiber-rich food sources will help you keep your hunger and cravings at bay.

Since fiber isn't exactly the quickest to digest, it will ensure that you continue to feel fuller for longer durations of time. Furthermore, fiber ensures that our blood sugar levels are regulated, another benefit that may help many, especially diabetic patients.

Stay Hydrated

It goes without saying that we need water to survive, and regardless of what diet you choose to carry on with, nothing changes the importance of water. I have seen many people who take up the sugar-free diet challenge and find themselves in troubling situations. Upon closer inspection, I learned that these people overlooked the importance of water and were only drinking a couple of glasses of water a day.

To ensure that you do not run into unnecessary issues and to ensure that your overall health remains good, drink as much water as possible. It is recommended that you drink around eight glasses of water a day. That will help you to manage your blood sugar levels, and it will help curb your sugar cravings as well.

It is also important to mention that drinking water will allow for better bowel movement as well. Couple this with protein and fiber, and you end up with a perfect balance of almost everything you need in a day.

Artificial Sweeteners Stay Out

Do not fall for the so-called "safe" and "healthy" gimmicks which many artificial sweeteners use on their packaging. These should remain out of our diets for life. When consumed, they will derail us from our primary goal.

There is research that suggests that using artificial sweeteners impacts our metabolic rate. As a result, this increases our cravings, pushing us to consume more food, which may eventually lead to weight gain, all of which are the things we are trying to avoid in the first place.

Manage Stress Effectively

Stress will follow you around, even when you are home and are trying to sleep. Unfortunately, there aren't any sure-fire ways to permanently eliminate stress. There are, however, some effective ways through which you can reduce and manage your stress.

You can search for simple meditation techniques, various breathing exercises, and some other forms of self-hypnosis. These are great, and most of these can be done in any setting. You will only need around 10 minutes of your time, but the impact that these techniques will have are well worth those 10 minutes.

It is a good idea to pick up on some stress relieving exercises because as soon as you show sugar the door, stress will start building up quicker than you might imagine. Prolonged stress can further cause mental, emotional, and overall health-related problems.

Exercise

One of the finest ways to divert your mind and feel fresh is to exercise. When you start a diet and your body experiences symptoms, exercise can help you to forget all about these adverse effects.

Besides, exercise is a wonderful way to promote healthy living. Whether you prefer to run, lift weights, or do gymnastics, exercise can certainly provide you with an improved mood, better health, improved sleep habits, and so much more.

Before you do go out and exercise, it is a good idea to consult your doctor first, especially if you are suffering from underlying issues such as heart problems, asthma, or any other ailment which may cause issues.

Quality Over Quantity

A lot of people tend to focus on the quantity of the food they consume, which is what normally leaves them without results. When you start focusing on the quality instead, you not only gain health benefits, but you will also find your withdrawal symptoms easing up by a significant amount.

A good way to up your food quality is to reduce high-sugar food items and replace them with nutrient-dense food items, such as fish, beans, or vegetables of your choice. Another good way would be to add some supplements such as Vitamin B, C, and magnesium. All of these combined will ensure that your symptoms are more manageable and that you continue to gain the best health benefits possible as you proceed with your diet.

Sleep

This one is fairly easy; get your eight hours a day. However, problems may occur if your symptoms are not letting you sleep peacefully. For that, exercise and meditation may come in handy.

If you work out during the day or the evening, your sleep at night will improve automatically. Same goes good with meditation. Although you do not get as many physical benefits as you would normally feel with exercise, you will, however, experience almost the same mental and emotional benefits. These boosts will automatically promote good sleep and will ensure that you continue to sleep undisturbed.

You need your sleep to ensure that your body gets its time to rejuvenate and be ready to take on the next day's challenges. Always make sure that you do whatever is necessary to get some well-deserved sleep.

Motivate Yourself

It would certainly be nice if others around you did this part, but instead of taking that chance, it is a good idea to start encouraging and motivating yourself. Every day, let yourself know that you are doing a brilliant job. If you managed to go through a day without sugar, you can make it another day. After the next one, let yourself know that you can go further. Before you know it, you will be ending your three weeks' long journey on a high note.

It is also a good idea to tune into some motivational stories you may find on the internet. These can often provide you with the inspiration and motivation you need to keep on going. The cravings will become a thing of the past, and you will continue to look forward to a new day's challenge, with positivity and determination.

Some Additional Tips

This is the last section of the first part of the book and a good time to share some additional tips that will help you in your three weeks' long journey, and more.

- Start by removing the sweet stuff from your life. It may be a bit tricky, but to help you clear out the high-sugar products, create a list of items which you would normally consume. Include everything, from sugary drinks to alcohol, juices, snack bars, chocolate, and so on. Make it a goal to delete everything from the list after having reduced the availability of these items in your home significantly. It would be ideal to permanently remove some of these sugary sources for good.
- Make it a point in life that you will no longer fall for the "healthy" label trap. Stop buying items which have

hidden sugar content as they can easily derail you from your sugar-free quest. Some common items to watch out for include:

- fruit muesli
- fruit juices
- sugary yogurt
- sugary health bars
- Always look at the labels. Previously, we learned what to look out for in labels and how to read them correctly. Use all that you have learned and ensure that you always know what product you are about to buy. If it contains hidden or additional sugar, let it remain on the shelf.
- Low-fat food items are generally loaded with sugar. Be sure to check labels, if applicable. Otherwise, it's a good idea to research these products before purchasing them. A good alternate would be to search for items with high fiber and low sugar.
- Get creative in the kitchen and come up with your own dressings for salads. The ones which are available in the supermarket are generally full of sugar. It is fairly easy to make dressings at home, all you need are the right ingredients. It may take a few tries, but once you learn how to make dressing, you will never need to rely on buying it from the store ever again.
- Say goodbye to the sugar you bought from the store. You will no longer be needing that. Instead, rely on

naturally occurring sweet ingredients, and use those as a good replacement. Not only are they healthy, but they may very well be cheaper as well.

- This book has provided you with almost a complete plan. I say almost because a part of it is yet to come. Use this plan to ensure you know what to do and what to expect and then plan accordingly.

- There is no point in waiting for the "right time" as that will never come. There is no better time than now, and if you cannot start now, you cannot start at all. Do not wait or give yourself a starting date. Instead, let yourself know that this new change begins now.

- If your pantry is already restocked, use the next section of the book to look out for some good recipes. If you like a recipe or two, use that as a starting point. However, if you are thinking of restocking your pantry, you may want to go through the recipes first before going out to do your shopping.

And that brings us to the end of this part of the book. We are done with all the theories, all the science, all the tips and tricks of the game. It is now time to begin what you really came here to learn. It is time to pick up the notebook and start noting down the recipes. In the next few chapters, I will provide you with numerous recipes for breakfast, lunch, dinner, and more. With that said, let's put on the apron, and let's start teasing our taste buds for a change.

5

BREAKFAST

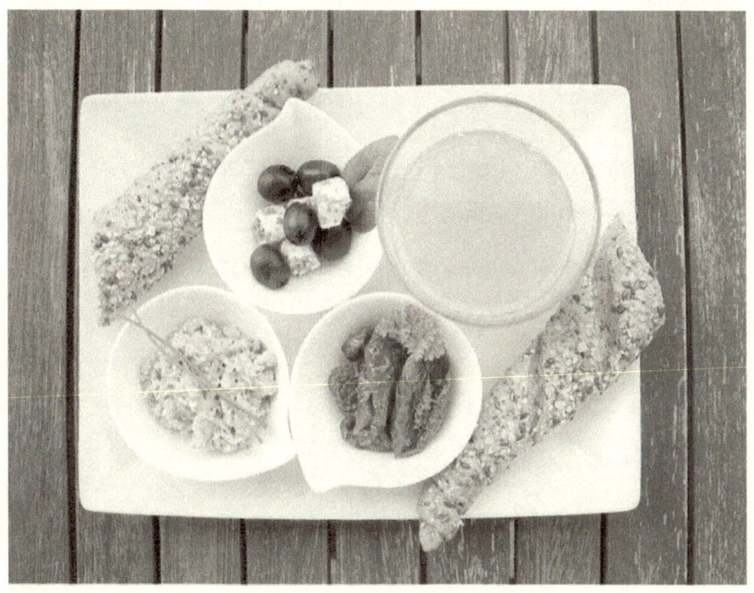

F inally, we have arrived at the part which we have all been waiting for far too long. Needless to say, the journey so far has been one of knowledge, information, and a bit of boredom as well, but that is all about to change.

The 21-day sugar-free diet is not exactly a diet if there is no actual cooking and preparation involved. The only reason this part came second was to ensure that you know some of the health-related jargon, some facts and figures, and some insight into the science that is at play here. Now that you have a fair idea of what you might expect, it is time to get started.

From here on out, I will provide you with a number of different recipes for breakfast, lunch, and dinner. That is not all—I will also be providing you with some bonus recipes for sauces, dips, and snacks, just to ensure that this diet is neither dull nor boring.

To make the most of these recipes, you can choose to mix them for each day, giving yourself a treat, and something new to look forward to at every meal. How does that work? Here is a quick example:

Day One
Breakfast recipe # 4

Lunch recipe #9

Dinner recipe # 1

Day Two
Breakfast recipe # 8

Lunch recipe #3

Dinner recipe #2

You are completely free to choose which recipes go where. The idea is to ensure that you get to enjoy a variety of flavors with every single meal.

You do not necessarily have to follow the recipes to the dot. As long as you have the information from the previous chapter, you can always modify some ingredients to make the recipe unique and more to your liking. All you need to do is to ensure that whatever you choose to substitute, it falls in the same GI ranking region as the ingredient you may be replacing it with. This will limit the sugar intake to roughly the same quantity or less. If the sugar quantity or the GI rank is higher, it is best to avoid that ingredient and replace it with another one with a relatively lower GI score.

If you cannot recall what GI scores are, we discussed the Glycemic Index in Chapter 3. You can always refer to that as a source of inspiration and ideas. You can also browse the internet and search for a complete list of food items with their relative GI rankings. This will provide you with a clear picture of the kind of food items you are using and which ones may be a better choice for a specific recipe that you want to try.

It greatly helps if you can write that list down, or simply print it and keep it nearby. It will always be there for you when you need to refer to it, saving you time and energy when deciding about the food items you should be using. With that said, let us get started with the recipes.

RECIPES FOR BREAKFAST

Breakfast is the most important meal of the day. Get this right, and you will have enough energy to go through the rest of the day with ease. In this section, I will provide you with some of the most mouth-watering breakfast recipes, all aimed to ensure that you keep your sugar levels to a bare minimum while enjoying exquisite tastes.

Note: Recipes retrieved from Clean Eating Magazine (https://www.cleaneatingmag.com/)

Mediterranean Veggie Toast

Prep time: 10 minutes

Duration: 25 minutes

Servings: Two

Nutritional Facts

Serving size: One toast with topping

Calories: 304

Carbohydrate content: 26 grams

Cholesterol: 32 milligrams

Fat content: 16 grams

Fiber content: 6 grams

Protein content: 15 grams

Saturated fats: 7 grams

Sodium content: 573 milligrams

Sugar content: 5 grams

Monounsaturated fat: 6 grams

Polyunsaturated fat: 2 grams

Ingredients

- 1/2 cup of zucchini, thinly sliced
- 1/4 teaspoon of sea salt
- 1/2 cup of whole-milk ricotta cheese
- 2 tablespoons of all-natural pesto (prepared)
- 2 slices of whole-grain bread
- 2 roma tomatoes, sliced
- 2 white mushrooms, sliced thinly
- 1/4 teaspoon of dried oregano

Preparation

1. Spread the zucchini on some paper towel. Sprinkle these with salt. Allow them to remain there for 8 to 10 minutes, until softened. Use another paper towel to dry them.
2. Stir ricotta with pesto in a small bowl and set it aside.
3. Using a toaster oven, toast the bread on the rack until it just starts turning golden. Transfer the bread on to a small baking tray. This is usually the tray that comes with the oven. Set your toaster oven to 375 degrees.
4. Spread the ricotta mixture on top of the toast. Layer

the tomato, zucchini, and mushrooms on top in any order. Sprinkle with some oregano. Bake these until the ricotta is properly warmed through. The veggies should be light brown. This should take no more than 10 minutes.

White Beans and Roasted Red Pepper Toast

Prep time: 15 minutes

Duration: 15 minutes

Servings: Four

Nutritional Facts

Serving size: One toast with some bean spread and avocado

Calories: 405

Carbohydrate content: 48 grams

Fat content: 18 grams

Fiber content: 14 grams

Protein content: 16 grams

Saturated fat: 3 grams

Sodium content: 316 milligrams

Sugar content: 3 grams

Monounsaturated fat: 12 grams

Polyunsaturated fat: 3 grams

Ingredients

- 2 cups of unsalted white beans, rinsed and drained
- 1 small and roasted red pepper, drained
- 1 tablespoon of olive oil (additional for drizzling)
- 1 clove of garlic (optional)
- 1/4 teaspoon of sea salt
- Pinch of red pepper flakes
- 4 slices of whole-grain bread
- 2 small avocados, peeled, pitted and sliced thinly

Preparation

1. Use a food processor and combine red peppers, beans, garlic, oil, salt, and pepper flakes. Process these until the mixture is smooth and creamy.
2. Just before serving, toast the bread. Spread this mixture on the toast and top the toast with avocado. Drizzle some additional oil. Serve and enjoy!

Lumberjack Toast

Servings: Two

Nutritional Facts

Serving size: One slice

Calories: 365

Carbohydrate content: 29 grams

Cholesterol content: 190 milligrams

Fat content: 23 grams

Fiber content: 10 grams

Protein content: 13 grams

Saturated fat: 5 grams

Sodium content: 334 milligrams

Sugar content: 5 grams

Monounsaturated fat: 12 grams

Polyunsaturated fat: 3 grams

Ingredients

- 1/2 sweet potato, cut crosswise (¼- inch rounds), peeled
- 2 teaspoons of olive oil or ghee
- 2 large eggs
- 2 slices of whole-grain bread
- 1 peeled avocado, pitted and sliced thinly
- 2 tablespoons of red onion, finely chopped
- 1/8 teaspoon of sea salt
- All-natural hot sauce

Preparation

1. Begin by preheating the oven to 400 degrees. Use a parchment-lined baking sheet and arrange the potatoes

in a single line. Use a cooking spray and mist on either side. Bake these until they turn light golden in color, turning halfway. This should take around 20 to 25 minutes.

2. Heat some olive oil or ghee in a medium skillet over medium flame. Crack one egg in a small bowl, and then slide it into the skillet. Do the same for the remainder of the eggs. Cook these until the whites are done and the yolk is to your desired doneness.

3. Toast the bread. Divide the potatoes, avocado, eggs, salt, onion, and the hot sauce evenly on the toasts. Serve.

Surfer Toast

Servings: Two

Nutritional Facts

Serving size: One slice

Calories: 345

Carbohydrate content: 33 grams

Cholesterol content: 10 milligrams

Fat content: 3 grams

Protein content: 16 grams

Saturated fat: 3 grams

Sodium content: 471 milligrams

Sugar content: 7 grams

Monounsaturated fat: 11 grams

Polyunsaturated fat: 3 grams

Ingredients

- 1 peeled avocado, pitted and sliced thinly
- 2 slices of whole-grain bread, toasted
- 5 to 6 grape tomatoes, halved
- 2 ounces of smoked wild salmon
- 1/3 cup sprouts or any microgreen of your choice
- 1 tablespoon of fresh dill, with the tougher stems removed

Preparation

1. Smash the avocado with a fork inside a bowl. Spread it on the toast.
2. Top each of the toast pieces with half of the tomatoes, salmon, dill, and sprouts.

The Hipster (Mushrooms, Gruyere, and Truffle Oil)

Servings: Two

Nutritional Facts

Serving size: One slice

Calories: 237

Carbohydrate content: 21.5 grams

Cholesterol content: 16 milligrams

Fat content: 13 grams

Fiber content: 3 grams

Protein content: 10 grams

Saturated fat: 4 grams

Sodium content: 398 milligrams

Sugar content: 5 grams

Monounsaturated fat: 7 grams

Polyunsaturated fat: 2 grams

Ingredients

- 2 slices of whole-grain peasant bread (seeded)
- 1 clove of garlic
- 1 ounce of Gruyere cheese, shredded
- 2 teaspoons of olive oil
- 1 cup of mixed Japanese mushrooms
- 1/8 teaspoon of sea salt
- 1/2 teaspoon of all-natural truffle oil
- 1/2 teaspoon of chopped chives

Preparation

1. Begin by preheating a grill to medium. First, grill the bread until it is lightly toasted and shows light grill

marks. This is generally two minutes on each side. Alternatively, you can use a toaster.

2. Using the end of the garlic clove, cut a thin slice off. With the cut side, rub one side of the bread.

3. Put the cheese on the toast and place it under the broiler until it is melted. This may take between 30 to 60 seconds.

4. Heat the olive oil in a medium skillet over medium flame. Add in the mushrooms and cook these for two to three minutes until they are golden brown from underneath. Season these with salt and sauté for three to four minutes until these are softened.

5. Top the toasts with the sautéed mushrooms. Finally, drizzle truffle oil and then top that with chives. Serve.

Baked Brie on Toasted Baguette

Prep Time: 10 minutes

Duration: 25 minutes

Servings: Eight

Nutritional Facts

Serving size: 2-inch wedge brie, 1/4 cup of toppings, and 3 toasts

Calories: 226

Carbohydrate content: 25 grams

Cholesterol content: 28 milligrams

Fat contents: 11 grams

Fiber content: 2.5 grams

Protein content: 10 grams

Saturated fat: 5 grams

Sodium content: 333 milligrams

Sugar content: 9 grams

Polyunsaturated fat: 1 gram

Ingredients

- 3 tablespoons of raw honey
- 3/4 teaspoon of dried lavender
- 1/2 pound strawberries, cored, stemmed, and chopped
- 8 ounces of round brie cheese
- 8 ounces of whole-wheat baguette, thin sliced (half of a large loaf)
- 1/3 cup of roasted shelled pistachios, unsalted and chopped

Preparation

1. In the lower-middle and the upper-middle positions of the oven, arrange the racks. Preheat to around 375 degrees. Use a small saucepan on medium-high heat, and add in honey, lavender, and two teaspoons of water. Now, bring it to a simmer while stirring frequently. Reduce the heat to low and simmer until

fragrant. Use a medium bowl and add strawberries and honey syrup. Stir to combine these and then set aside.

2. Use a medium-rimmed baking sheet and line it with a nonstick foil or parchment paper. Next, place the cheese in the center. Bake using the upper rack until the cheese starts to feel very soft when pressed. This should take around 15 to 17 minutes.

3. Using a large-rimmed baking sheet, place the baguette slices and use the lower rack to bake until lightly toasted. Now, transfer the cheese to a serving plate. Using a knife, cut a thin wedge to allow the cheese to ooze out. Top it with strawberries and the syrup, add pistachios and serve with baguette slices.

Smoked Trout Salad

Prep Time: 25 minutes

Duration: 25 minutes

Servings: Four

Nutritional Facts

Serving size: 1/4 of recipe

Calories: 324

Carbohydrate content: 16 grams

Cholesterol content: 69 milligrams

Fat content: 19 grams

Fiber content: 6 grams

Protein content: 24 grams

Saturated fat: 4 grams

Sodium content: 588 milligrams

Sugar content: 8 grams

Monounsaturated fat: 8 grams

Polyunsaturated fat: 4 grams

Ingredients

Dressing

- 1/3 cup of full-fat sour cream
- 1/4 cup of fresh dill, chopped
- 1/2 teaspoon of lemon zest and 3 tablespoons of lemon juice
- 2 teaspoons of Dijon mustard
- 1/4 teaspoon of sea salt and black pepper each

Salad

- 1 large grapefruit
- 5 cups of torn butter lettuce
- 8 ounces of smoked trout
- 2 large stalks celery, sliced thinly
- 1 avocado, pitted, peeled, and sliced
- 1/2 red onion, either sliced or pickled
- 2 tablespoons of roasted and salted sunflower seeds

Preparation

1. Prepare the dressing. Use a small bowl and whisk together all the dressing ingredients.
2. Prepare the salad. Cut thin slices from the top and bottom of the grapefruit. Start from the top and cut the peels and pith away. Turn it sideways and slice the grapefruit into wheels.
3. Divide the trout, lettuce, grapefruit, avocado, celery, and onion among plates. Top each of these with dressing and the seeds. Serve.

Fruits and Oats Salad with Prosciutto

Prep Time: 25 minutes

Duration: 40 minutes

Servings: Four

Nutritional Facts

Serving size: 1/4 of the recipe

Calories: 284

Carbohydrate content: 16 grams

Cholesterol content: 19 milligrams

Fat content: 21 grams

Fiber content: 3 grams

Protein content: 10 grams

Saturated fat: 5 grams

Sodium content: 678 milligrams

Sugar content: 9 grams

Monounsaturated fat: 12 grams

Polyunsaturated fat: 4 grams

Ingredients

- 2 ounces of sliced prosciutto
- 1/4 cup of extra virgin olive oil, divided
- 1/3 cup of rolled oats
- 2 tablespoons of finely chopped walnuts, unsalted
- 1 teaspoon of raw honey
- 1/4 teaspoon of chopped fresh thyme
- 1/2 teaspoon of sea salt, divided
- 1/2 teaspoon of ground black pepper
- 2 oranges
- 1 tablespoon of red wine vinegar
- 4 cups of baby arugula
- 2 ounces of soft goat cheese
- Balsamic glaze (this is optional)

Preparation

1. Start by preheating the oven to 350 degrees. Line a large baking sheet with parchment paper. Lay the prosciutto on the sheet, and leave some space between each slice. Bake these until they are crisp (around 12 to

16 minutes). Be sure to watch these to prevent overbrowning. Transfer these to a rack and allow them to cool completely.

2. In the meantime, heat one quarter of the oil in a medium skillet on medium heat. Add in the oats, honey, thyme, and walnuts. Sprinkle in about 1/2 of the salt and pepper and continue cooking. Stir and shake the pan often until they are fragrant and changing color to golden. This should not take more than six minutes. Transfer these to a bowl and let them cool.

3. Cut off the top and bottom of an orange. Slice the peel and pith off, working from top to bottom. Cut between the membranes to allow segments to be released. Remove the segment while reserving the juice that may come out. Squeeze the juice out from the remainder of the oranges in a bowl.

4. Add the remainder of oil, Dijon, vinegar, and the remaining half of salt and pepper.

5. Divide the arugula among the plates. Next, crumble the cheese on top. Divide the orange segments among salads. Then, top these with oat mixture and the prosciutto. If using glaze, drizzle that now. Serve.

Mediterranean Salad With a Twist

Prep Time: 20 minutes

Duration: 50 minutes

Servings: Four

Nutritional Facts

Serving size: 1/4 of the recipe

Calories: 534

Carbohydrate content: 27 grams

Cholesterol content: 199 milligrams

Fat content: 41 grams

Fiber content: 9 grams

Protein content: 17 grams

Saturated fat: 8 grams

Sodium content: 681 milligrams

Sugar content: 8 grams

Monounsaturated fat: 26.5 grams

Polyunsaturated fat: 4.5 grams

Ingredients

Vinaigrette

- 1/2 cup of extra virgin olive oil
- 2 cloves of garlic, minced
- 3 tablespoons of fresh parsley, chopped
- 2 tablespoons of fresh mint, chopped

- 1 tablespoon of fresh basil, chopped
- 1 tablespoon of chopped chives
- 1/4 cup of white wine vinegar
- 1 teaspoon of Dijon mustard
- 1/2 teaspoon of sea salt
- 1/4 teaspoon of ground black pepper

Salad

- 1 15-ounce can of chickpeas, rinsed, drained and dried thoroughly
- 2 teaspoons of extra virgin olive oil
- Sea salt
- 1 head romaine lettuce, chopped
- 1 English cucumber, chopped and quartered lengthwise
- 8 ounces of grape or cherry tomatoes, halved
- 2 ounces of full-fat feta cheese, crumbled
- 1/2 cup of prepared hummus (this is optional)
- 4 large hard-boiled eggs, halved lengthwise
- Ground black pepper

Preparation

1. Start by making the vinaigrette. Combine 1/2 of garlic and olive oil in a small skillet over low heat. Heat these until the mixture starts to sizzle. Allow it to sizzle for

30 seconds before transferring it to a small bowl. Let it cool off. Combine the remaining 1/2 of oil, mint, basil, parsley, mustard, and vinegar in a small food processor. Use the pulse system to mix. Add the cooled garlic mixture along with salt and pepper. Blend these until they are well combined.

2. Preparing the salad: preheat the oven to 350 degrees. In a regular bowl, toss the chickpeas with salt and oil. Then, spread these on a baking sheet. Bake these for 40 to 45 minutes until they are very crisp and golden. Shake the pan occasionally. Once done, transfer these to a bowl and let them cool.

3. Combine cucumber, romaine, feta, and tomatoes in a bowl. Use enough dressing to coat these lightly. If needed, add more dressing. Spread the hummus on the bottom of each plate. Top these with the cucumber mixture. Place the two egg halves on each of the plates and sprinkle additional salt. Season the salads with pepper, and finally sprinkle the crispy chickpeas.

Smoked Salmon Omelette

Prep time: 15 minutes

Duration: 25 minutes

Servings: Four

Nutritional Facts

Serving size: One omelette

Calories: 381

Carbohydrate content: 6.5 grams

Cholesterol content: 412 milligrams

Fat content: 27 grams

Fiber content: 1 gram

Protein content: 27 grams

Saturated fat: 12 grams

Sodium content: 714 milligrams

Sugar content: 5 grams

Monounsaturated fat: 10 grams

Polyunsaturated fat: 3 grams

Ingredients

- 1 red beet, peeled
- 1 1/2 tablespoons of balsamic vinegar
- 1 tablespoon of olive oil
- 1 tablespoon and an additional 2 teaspoons of finely chopped chives
- 1 tablespoon of fresh dill, finely chopped and divided
- 1/2 teaspoon of organic cane sugar
- Kosher salt, black pepper (to taste)
- 8 large eggs
- 1/4 cup of whole milk
- 2 tablespoons of organic, unsalted butter

- 6 ounces of smoked salmon
- 4 ounces of goat cheese, fresh

Preparation

1. Start with the beet relish: use a box grater and coarsely grate the beet in a medium bowl. Add in the oil, vinegar, 2 teaspoons of chives, dill, and the cane juice and stir. Season the mixture with salt and pepper to taste and then set it aside.

2. Using a large bowl, whisk eggs and milk together, and blend them nicely. Season the mixture with salt.

3. Put a medium nonstick skillet on medium-low heat. Add 1/2 tablespoon of butter. Swirl it to coat the skillet. Pour 1/4 of the egg mixture. Swirl it in the pan to ensure even coating. Cook and then lift the edges using a silicone spatula. Allow the uncooked eggs to run right into the pan. This should be done for about two minutes or at least until most of the egg is settled but the omelette is still runny at the top. Now, arrange 1/4 of the smoked salmon on top of the omelette. Top this with 1/4 of cheese, scatter 1 1/2 tablespoons of the beet relish on top. Fold the omelette and transfer it to a plate. Repeat the same and make three more.

4. Finally, sprinkle the omelettes with the remaining tablespoon of chives, and one teaspoon of dill. Serve with remaining beet relish.

6

LUNCH

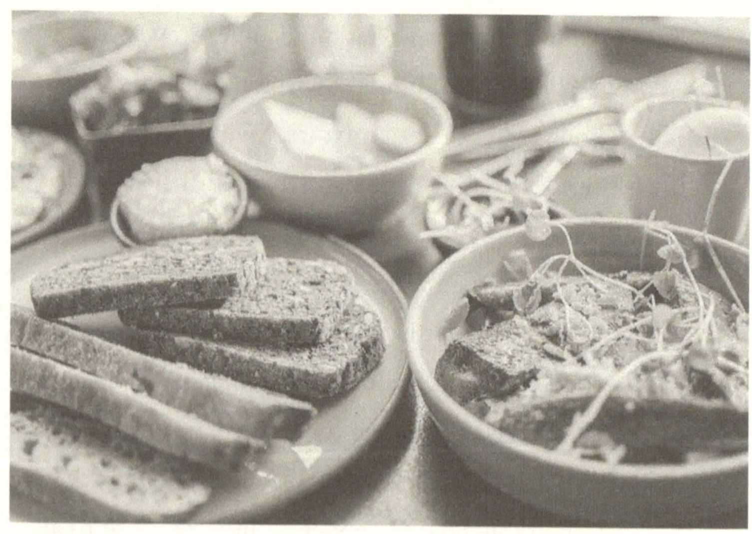

Just like a good breakfast, lunch is equally important. To ensure that we continue with the momentum, let us look at some mouth-watering recipes for our lunch.

THE LUNCH RECIPES

Sweet & Sour Chicken Wrap with Almond and Ginger Sauce

Prep time: 20 minutes

Duration: 80 minutes

Serves: Four

Nutritional Facts

Serving size: One-fourth of the recipe

Calories: 342

Carbohydrate content: 13 grams

Cholesterol content: 60 milligrams

Fat content: 20 grams

Fiber content: 5 grams

Protein content: 28 grams

Saturated fat: 2 grams

Sodium content: 482 milligrams

Sugar content: 6 grams

Monounsaturated fat: 11 grams

Polyunsaturated fat: 5 grams

Ingredients

Rolls

- 2 carrots, cut into the shape of matchsticks
- 1 cup of rice vinegar
- 3 tablespoons of organic sugar
- 1 teaspoon of sea salt
- 2 cups of shredded or sliced, cooked chicken breast
- 2 cups of finely shredded purple cabbage or Napa cabbage
- 1/2 of a small English cucumber, cut into matchsticks
- 1/4 cup of fresh mint, basil leaves, each
- 16 leaves of Bibb lettuce (around 2 heads)

Sauce

- 1 tablespoon of avocado oil
- 2 cloves of garlic
- 2 teaspoons of peeled garlic, minced
- 1/3 cup of creamy almond butter
- 2 tablespoons of coconut aminos
- 1 tablespoon of rice vinegar
- 2 teaspoons of toasted sesame oil
- 1 teaspoon of fish sauce
- 1 to 2 teaspoons of sriracha (this is optional)
- Sea salt to taste

Preparation

1. Begin by pickling carrots for filling: place the carrots in a small bowl. Combine sugar, vinegar, and salt in a saucepan. Bring these to almost a boil, while stirring to dissolve the sugar and salt. Pour in the carrots. Let them cool by refrigerating them. This may take an hour, or you can make one day prior to cooking.

2. Make the sauce: add oil, ginger, and garlic to a small skillet on low heat. Cook these until they sizzle. Transfer these to a cup and let them cool. Get a small food processor, add in aminos, almond butter, sesame oil, vinegar, fish sauce, cooled garlic mixture and sriracha, and blend them until they are smooth. Add a little water at a time until the sauce has the desired consistency.

3. Assemble the wraps: begin by draining the carrot mixture. Transfer this to a bowl. Next, place chicken, cabbage, mint, basil, cucumber, and sauce in separate plates or bowls. Build the wraps using the lettuce leaves just before eating.

Chicken Banh Mi Sandwich

Prep time: 25 minutes
Duration: 55 minutes
Serves: Four

Nutritional Facts

Serving size: One sandwich

Calories: 266

Carbohydrate content: 42 grams

Cholesterol content: 31 milligrams

Fat content: 3 grams

Fiber content: 8 grams

Protein content: 21 grams

Sodium content: 425 milligrams

Sugar content: 5 grams

Ingredients

- 1/2 cup of rice vinegar
- 3 tablespoons of organic sugar
- 4 radishes, sliced thinly
- 2 green onions, sliced thinly
- 1 cup of savoy cabbage, sliced thinly
- 1 cup of julienned and peeled carrots
- 3/4 teaspoon of sea salt, divided
- 2 4-ounce boneless and skinless chicken breasts
- 1/2 teaspoon of fresh ground black pepper
- 4 whole-grain buns
- High-heat cooking oil
- 1 cup of fresh cilantro leaves

Preparation

1. Place a small saucepan over medium-high heat, bring 1/2 a cup of water, cane juice, and vinegar to boil. Once done, remove from the heat and transfer the contents to a heat-proof bowl. Allow it to cool for around five minutes. Then, add in radishes, cabbage, onions, carrots, and 1/2 teaspoon of salt. Cover and refrigerate for 30 minutes or more. You can also refrigerate this overnight.

2. In the meantime, season the chicken with the remaining 1/4 teaspoon of salt and pepper. Now, heat up a grill on medium high. Oil the grate lightly. Add in the chicken and grill it, turning it halfway, until it is lightly brown and is no longer pink. This should take around five to six minutes for each side. Transfer this to a cutting board and use foil to loosely cover it. Put the buns on the grill and toast.

3. Next, cut the chicken into thinner slices. Divide these slices among the buns. Use tongs and remove the vegetables from the vinegar mixture. Shake the vegetables slightly over the bowl to remove any excess liquid. Finally, divide these vegetables evenly and top them with cilantro.

Goat Cheese and Kalamata Panini

Prep time: 7 minutes

Duration: 11 minutes

Serves: Four

Nutritional Facts

Serving size: One sandwich

Calories: 301

Carbohydrate content: 50 grams

Cholesterol content: 6.5 milligrams

Fat content: 6 grams

Fiber content: 5 grams

Protein content: 9 grams

Saturated fat: 0.5 grams

Sodium content: 537 milligrams

Sugar content: 13 grams

Ingredients

- 14 pitted and chopped Kalamata olives
- 1/4 cup of chopped red onions
- 4 cloves of garlic, minced
- 2 teaspoons of dried basil
- 1/4 teaspoon of red pepper flakes
- 1 tablespoon of balsamic vinegar
- 1 12-ounce whole-grain Italian loaf of bread, halved

- 2 cups of baby spinach leaves
- 2 1/2-ounce pieces goat cheese crumbled
- 1 large tomato, sliced in 8 rounds
- Olive oil cooking spray

Preparation

1. Using a medium bowl, combine together olives, garlic, basil, onion, pepper flakes, and vinegar. Put the bread halves on a cutting board, and spoon in the olive mixture onto the bottom half of the bread (cut side up). Next, top this with spinach, tomato, and cheese. Then use the top of the bread and press down lightly. Use a serrated knife to cut bread into four equal pieces.

2. Heat up a large skillet on medium heat. Coat the skillet using the cooking spray and add in the sandwiches. Use aluminum foil to cover the sandwiches and then add weight by topping them with a dinner plate and some bread plates. Cook for the next two minutes until they are golden brown. Remove the plates and foil and flip the sandwich over. Once again, use the foil and plates to add weight. This time, reduce the heat to medium low and cook for another two minutes. Remove the sandwiches from heat and keep them covered for two more minutes. Serve.

Roast Pork and Nectarine Panini

Prep time: 55 minutes

Duration: 120 minutes

Serves: Four

Nutritional Facts

Serving size: One sandwich

Calories: 396

Carbohydrate content: 84 grams

Cholesterol content: 84 milligrams

Fat content: 6 grams

Fiber content: 6 grams

Protein content: 40 grams

Saturated fat: 2 grams

Sodium content: 476 milligrams

Sugar content: 18 grams

Polyunsaturated fat: 1 gram

Ingredients

- 1 pound of pork tenderloin
- Olive oil cooking spray
- 1 teaspoon of chile powder
- 1/2 teaspoon of dried oregano
- Ground black pepper to taste
- 8 1-ounce slices of whole-wheat bread
- 4 ounces of Swiss cheese, sliced thinly
- 2 nectarines, thinly sliced and pitted

- 3/4 cup of spinach leaves
- Tomato jam
- 1 pound of tomato, chopped
- 1/4 cup of raw honey
- 1/4 teaspoon of sea salt
- 2 tablespoons of apple cider vinegar
- 1/2 teaspoon of ground ginger

Preparation

1. Start by preparing the jam. Use a large saucepan to combine tomatoes, salt, and honey together. Using medium-high heat, bring this mixture to a simmer. Reduce the heat to medium low, and let it simmer until almost all of the juice is evaporated. Reduce the heat to low and cover the saucepan. Cook for another 25 minutes, stirring occasionally until the tomatoes soften. Add the ginger and vinegar and simmer without any cover for another 10 to 15 minutes until the mixture is slightly thick. Allow it to cool at room temperature for half an hour before using it.

2. Preheat the oven at 350 degrees. Coat a single baking sheet with cooking spray. Next, place the pork on the sheet and mist it with the spray. Season the sides with chile powder, pepper, and oregano. Roast this for around 25 minutes, until it is no longer pink. Let it rest for 10 minutes and then slice it thinly.

3. Use one ounce of cheese to top each of the four bread slices along with quarter of the pork, two tablespoons of jam, quarter of spinach, and quarter of nectarines. Place the remaining slices on top.

4. Preheat a panini press and coat it with cooking spray. Place the sandwiches on the cooking surface. Toast these until they are golden brown. Flip and repeat the process before serving.

French Grand Slam

Prep time: 20 minutes

Duration: 30 minutes

Serves: Two

Nutritional Facts

Serving size: One sandwich

Calories: 437

Carbohydrate content: 36 grams

Cholesterol content: 326 milligrams

Fat content: 19 grams

Protein content: 29 grams

Saturated fat: 7 grams

Sodium content: 652 milligrams

Sugar content: 14.5 grams

Polyunsaturated fat: 4 grams

Ingredients

- 3 large eggs, divided
- 1/2 cup milk
- 2 large egg whites
- 1 teaspoon of pure vanilla extract
- 4 slices of whole-grain bread
- Olive oil cooking spray
- 2 1-ounce slices of turkey bacon
- 2 tablespoons of cream cheese at room temperature
- 1 tablespoon of pure maple syrup
- 1 teaspoon of white vinegar

Preparation

1. Using a large bowl, mix together one whole egg, the egg whites, vanilla, and milk. Mist a large skillet with the cooking spray and heat it on medium-high heat. Dip the bread slices into the egg mixture and coat them well. Add the dipped slices to the skillet and cook until golden brown on both sides. Transfer them to a plate and cover them. Wipe the skillet clean and mist again with cooking spray, while using medium-high heat. Add in the bacon and cook until the bacon is crispy. Transfer this to a plate.

2. Using a small bowl, beat cream cheese and maple syrup

together with a spoon. Spread the mixture on two of the bread slices and top these with bacon.

3. Fill a medium pot with about three inches of water and heat it on medium. Add in vinegar and allow it to simmer gently. Crack open the remaining two eggs into two small bowls.

4. Using a wooden spoon, swirl the water and slip in the eggs carefully. Poach the eggs until the whites are set and the yolk remains runny. This should not take more than four minutes. Remove using a slotted spoon and drain the water completely. Place the eggs on top of the bacon and top that with remaining slices.

Connecticut-Style Lobster Rolls

Prep time: 15 minutes
Duration: 15 minutes
Serves: Four

Nutritional Facts

Serving size: One lobster roll
Calories: 335
Carbohydrate content: 27 grams
Cholesterol content: 188 milligrams
Fat content: 12 grams
Fiber content: 4 grams
Protein content: 29 grams

Saturated fat: 6 grams

Sodium content: 913 milligrams

Sugar content: 4 grams

Monounsaturated fat: 3 grams

Polyunsaturated fat: 2 grams

Ingredients

- 1 pound cooked lobster meat, chopped roughly, warmed
- 1/2 teaspoon of finely grated zest of lemon
- 3 tablespoon of lemon juice
- 1 teaspoon of paprika
- 1/4 teaspoon of sea salt, ground black pepper each
- 3 tablespoons of organic butter, unsalted
- 4 large Bibb lettuce leaves
- 4 whole-grain hotdog buns
- 1 tablespoon of fresh chives, chopped

Preparation

1. Using a bowl, combine together lobster, lemon juice and zest, paprika, and salt and pepper. Melt the butter and add it to the bowl and toss.
2. Divide the lobster mixture and lettuce among the buns. Sprinkle with chives and serve.

Chicken Salad Pesto Sandwich

Serves: Four

Ingredients

- 2 pounds of skinless, boneless chicken breasts
- 1/2 cup of finely chopped basil
- 1/4 cup of raw and unsalted walnuts
- 1 clove of garlic
- 1/4 cup of olive oil
- 1/4 cup of finely chopped red onion
- 1/4 teaspoon of lemon zest
- Juice from one lemon
- Salt and pepper, to taste
- 1 teaspoon of balsamic vinegar
- 8 slices of whole-grain bread
- 1/2 head of romaine lettuce

Preparation

1. Using a medium saucepan, poach the chicken breasts with a pinch of salt and just about enough water to cover the chicken. Bring this to a boil and then reduce the heat to simmer and cook. Cover the chicken as it cooks, until it is no longer pink. This should take around 10 minutes. Remove from heat, drain out all

the water, and shred the chicken. Use a fork to do the shredding.

2. Use a food processor to process chopped basil, walnuts, and garlic. Pulse until the mixture is finely chopped. Slow the motor down and add in 1/4 cup of olive oil. Blend well

3. Transfer the pesto to a larger bowl and add the shredded chicken along with 1/4 cup of chopped red onions, juice and zest of lemon, salt, and pepper.

4. Add balsamic vinegar and mix well to combine.

5. Toast the bread, and arrange four bread slices on a flat surface. Top each of the slices with chicken salad mixture. Then, divide the romaine lettuce on top. Top with the remaining four slices of bread.

Grilled Pear and Blue Cheese Sandwich

Prep time: 5 minutes

Duration: 7 minutes

Serves: One

Nutritional Facts

Serving size: One sandwich

Calories: 244

Carbohydrate content: 36 grams

Cholesterol content: 8 milligrams

Fat content: 5 grams

Fiber content: 6 grams

Protein content: 10.5 grams

Saturated fat: 2 grams

Sodium content: 302 milligrams

Sugar content: 13 grams

Ingredients

- 2 teaspoons of honey Dijon mustard
- 2 slices of whole-grain bread, divided
- 1/2 ounce of blue cheese, sliced
- 1/2 Anjou pear, sliced and cored
- 1/2f cup of baby arugula leaves

Preparation

1. Spread the Dijon on one slice of bread. Add cheese, arugula, and pear. Top with the remaining slice of bread. Place this sandwich in a hot panini press. Grill the sandwich until the cheese melts and starts to bubble. The bread should be crisp as well. This should only take around three minutes. Serve.

Spiced Egg Sandwich

Ingredients

- 2 eggs
- 1/4 cup of finely chopped celery
- 1 tablespoon of olive oil
- Pinch of cumin, salt, and pepper
- 2 slices of bread
- 2 lettuce leaves
- 2 slices of tomatoes

Preparation

1. Hard boil two eggs
2. Peel and then place the eggs in a bowl along with 1/4 cup of chopped celery, one tablespoon of olive oil, and a pinch of salt, pepper, and cumin each.
3. Mash these together and serve between two slices of bread with two lettuce leaves and tomatoes.

Veggie Pita Sandwich

Ingredients

- 1 1/2 tablespoons of olive tapenade
- 1 pita
- 1/2 cup of spinach

- 1/4 cup of chopped and roasted red bell pepper
- 2 tablespoons of cilantro
- 2 tablespoons of feta

Preparation

1. Spread 1 1/2 tablespoons of olive tapenade on a toasted pita. Top it with 1/2 cup of spinach, 1/4 cup of the chopped roasted red bell pepper, and two tablespoons of cilantro and feta. Serve.

DINNER

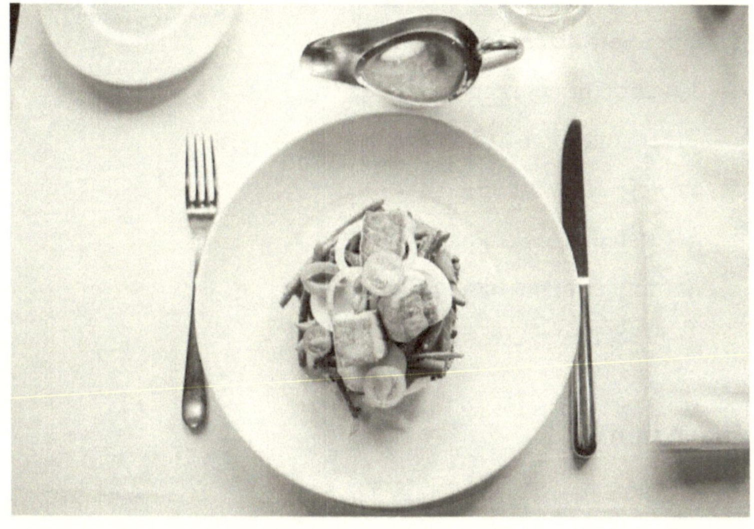

We began with breakfast, proceeded to lunch, and now it is time to look at some scrumptious dinner recipes!

DINNER RECIPES

Asian Chicken Salad Pita

Prep time: 20 minutes

Duration: 20 minutes

Serves: Four

Nutritional Facts

Serving size: One pita and 2/3 cups of filling

Calories: 374

Carbohydrate content: 41 grams

Cholesterol content: 72 milligrams

Fat content: 9 grams

Fiber content: 6 grams

Protein content: 35 grams

Saturated fat: 2 grams

Sodium content: 484 milligrams

Sugar content: 2 grams

Ingredients

- 2 tablespoons of natural cashew butter
- 2 tablespoons of chicken broth
- 1 tablespoon of apple cider vinegar
- 1 tablespoon of grated ginger
- 2 teaspoons of soy sauce

- 1/4 teaspoon of red pepper flakes
- 12-ounce cooked chicken breast, roughly chopped or shredded
- 2 scallions, sliced thinly
- 1 carrot, grated and peeled
- 1/2 cup of diced cucumber
- 2 tablespoons of freshly chopped cilantro leaves
- 4 whole-wheat pitas, spilt and halved

Preparation

1. Using a small bowl, whisk together cashew butter, vinegar, broth, soy sauce, ginger, and pepper flakes until the mixture is smooth. Set it aside.
2. Using a larger bowl, combine the chicken, carrots, scallions, cilantro, and cucumber. Add in the cashew mixture and stir. Fill each of the pita halves with chicken mixture. Serve.

Sautéed Salmon + Asian Marinade

Prep time: 15 minutes

Duration: 25 minutes (needs around one hour additional for marinating)

Serves: Two

Nutritional Facts

Serving size: 4-ounce piece of salmon

Calories: 230

Carbohydrate content: 9 grams

Cholesterol content: 62 milligrams

Fat content: 1 gram

Fiber content: 0.2 grams

Protein content: 24 grams

Saturated fat: 1 gram

Sodium content: 448 milligrams

Sugar content: 5 grams

Ingredients

- 2 cloves of garlic, chopped
- 1/4 cup of balsamic vinegar
- 2 tablespoons of soy sauce
- 2 teaspoons of olive oil cooking spray
- 1 tablespoon of chopped dill
- Juice from 1/2 a lemon
- 1/8 teaspoon of black pepper
- 2 4-ounce boneless salmon fillets, with or without skin

Preparation

1. Get a large baking dish or a resealable plastic bag. Put
   in garlic, soy sauce, vinegar, two teaspoons of oil,

lemon juice, dill, and pepper. Add the salmon and coat with mixture.

2. Marinate this at room temperature for an hour. Ensure that the salmon is fully immersed, otherwise you will need to turn it halfway through.

3. Use a large skillet and mist it with cooking spray. Heat on medium high. Add in the salmon and left-over marinade. Cook the salmon for six to eight minutes until it is easily flaked with a fork. If the salmon darkens quickly, lower the heat. Serve.

Asian Soba Salad and Lime Steak

Prep time: 15 minutes

Duration: 30 minutes

Serves: Four

Nutritional Facts

Serving size: 1 cup

Calories: 401

Carbohydrate content: 55 grams

Cholesterol content: 28 milligrams

Fat content: 9 grams

Fiber content: 7 grams

Protein content: 23 grams

Saturated fat: 2 grams

Sodium content: 498 milligrams

Sugar content: 8 grams

Polyunsaturated fat: 1 gram

Ingredients

- 2 scallions, with white and green parts separated, divided
- Juice from 1 lime
- 3 tablespoons of soy sauce, divided
- 1 teaspoon of sesame oil, divided
- 8-ounce flank steak or top sirloin, thinly sliced and trimmed
- 8-ounce Soba noodles
- 1 cup of frozen and shelled edamame
- 1/4 cup of brown rice vinegar
- 1 teaspoon of minced ginger
- 1 teaspoon of olive oil
- 2 red bell peppers, thinly sliced and seeded
- 8 ounces romaine lettuce, in bite-sized pieces

Preparation

1. Use a medium bowl to combine together white or light green parts of scallions, one teaspoon of soy sauce, lime juice, and half teaspoon of sesame oil. Add in the steak, toss this to coat, and marinate for around 10 minutes.

2. Bring a medium pot of water to boil. Add in noodles and edamame, and cook for about 10 minutes, right until the noodles are al dente. In the meantime, whisk ginger, vinegar, the remaining 2 tablespoons of soy sauce, and 1/2 teaspoon of sesame oil in a small bowl, and set it aside. Drain the noodles and edamame thoroughly. Use cold water to rinse. Return the edamame and noodles to the pot. Add in vinegar mixture and combine by tossing.

3. Using a large skillet on medium-high heat, heat olive oil. Transfer the steak to the skillet while discarding the marinade. Add in the peppers and sauté. Stir occasionally until the steak is cooked through.

4. Divide the noodle-edamame, lettuce, and the steak-pepper mixtures among plates. Garnish each with the reserved darker parts of scallion.

Five-Spice Pork Chili

Prep time: 45 minutes

Duration: 110 minutes

Serves: Six

Nutritional Facts

Serving size: 1 1/2 cups

Calories: 367

Carbohydrate content: 37 grams

Cholesterol content: 75 milligrams

Fat content: 5 grams

Fiber content: 8 grams

Protein content: 43 grams

Saturated fat: 2 grams

Sodium content: 203 milligrams

Sugar content: 6 grams

Ingredients

- 1/2 cup of dried wood ear fungus (optional, but worth it)
- 1 1/4 pound of lean ground pork or turkey
- 1 1/4 cups of dried black beans (soak these in water 24 hours prior to use or boil for at least an hour until al dente, drain, and then set aside)
- 3 cloves of garlic, chopped coarsely
- 1 small hot Thai red chile, chopped
- 2-inch piece of ginger, minced
- 1 teaspoon of Chinese five-spice powder
- 15 Chinese long beans, cut and trimmed into thirds
- 1 cup of stemmed, sliced shiitake mushrooms
- 1e teaspoon of toasted sesame oil
- 4 cups of chicken broth
- 4 cups of baby bok choy, rinsed, trimmed, and drained
- Sea salt and ground black pepper
- 5 green onions with white and green parts chopped

Preparation

1. If you intend to use the wood ear fungus, get a kettle of water and bring it to a boil. Use a small, heat-proof bowl, add in the wood ear, and cover with the boiling water. Soak it for around 10 minutes until it is soft. Drain the water and set it aside.

2. Mist a large and heavy-bottomed stock pot with cooking spray. Heat this on medium. Add the pork, stir, and continue breaking it up using a wooden spoon for eight to 10 minutes. Stop when it is browned.

3. Add in the wood ear, garlic, black beans, ginger, chile, and five-spice powder and continue to cook it. Stir constantly for around five minutes. Add the long beans, sesame oil, mushrooms, and the broth. Bring this mixture to a boil and then cover it while reducing the heat to medium low. Allow it to simmer for an hour. Before serving, add in the bok choy and simmer for another minute until it is just wilted. Season this with some salt and pepper and garnish with green onions.

Furikake Tuna Poke

Serves: Four

Nutritional Facts

Serving size: 1/4 of recipe

Calories: 439

Carbohydrate content: 55 grams

Cholesterol content: 34 milligrams

Fat content: 15 grams

Fiber content: 5 grams

Protein content: 28 grams

Saturated fat: 2 grams

Sodium content: 348 milligrams

Sugar content: 9 grams

Monounsaturated fat: 6 grams

Polyunsaturated fat: 6 grams

Ingredients

- 1 small daikon radish, thinly sliced
- 1/2 cup and 1 additional tablespoon of rice vinegar, divided
- 3 tablespoons of raw honey
- 3 tablespoons of sesame oil
- 1 tablespoon of tamari
- 1 clove of garlic, minced

- 1/4 cup of brown or black sesame seeds
- 2 to 3 large sheets of toasted nori, ground
- 1/4 cup of bonito flakes
- 1/2 teaspoon of sea salt
- Pinch of cayenne pepper (optional)
- 12-ounce sushi or sashimi grade tuna, cut in chunks
- 3 cups of cooked rice ramen noodles
- 1 large carrot, shredded
- 1 red onion, sliced thinly
- 1 cup of snow peas, sliced thinly
- 4 large red radishes, sliced thinly

Preparation

1. Pack the daikon in a glass pint jar. Use a small pot to bring half a cup of vinegar to boil. Remove it from heat and add honey. Stir it to dissolve. Pour over the daikon and then cover it for one to two hours. You can also refrigerate overnight.

2. Use a small bowl to whisk together tamari, oil, garlic, and the remaining tablespoon of vinegar. Set this aside.

3. Prepare the furikake. Using a small jar, add together nori, sesame seeds, salt, pepper, and bonito. Add in cayenne, if you are using it. Cover this and shake it. Pour the furikake into a shallow dish and dredge the tuna cubes in the mixture. You can now discard the excess furikake.

4. Assemble the bowls. Toss the noodles with half of the dressing. Divide between four bowls. Top each of the bowls using carrots, snow peas, onions, and radishes. Drizzle with the remaining dressing. Divide the pickled daikon and the tuna between bowls.

Sesame Pork Noodles with Bok Choy

Prep time: 15 minutes

Duration: 35 minutes

Serves: Four

Nutritional Facts

Serving size: 12 ounces

Calories: 405

Carbohydrate content: 55 grams

Cholesterol content: 143 milligrams

Fat content: 10 grams

Fiber content: 12 grams

Protein content: 28 grams

Saturated fat: 2 grams

Sodium content: 248 milligrams

Sugar content: 5 grams

Monounsaturated fat: 4 grams

Polyunsaturated fat: 3 grams

Ingredients

- 8 ounces of whole-grain spaghetti
- 1 tablespoon of sesame oil, divided
- 1/2 pound of pork tenderloin, sliced and trimmed into 1/4-inch thick strips
- 1 pound bok choy, remove stem ends, stems and leaves chopped roughly
- 4 cloves of garlic, sliced thinly
- 3 green onions, sliced
- 1 tablespoon of soy sauce
- 1 teaspoon of ground ginger
- 1/4 teaspoon of black pepper
- 1 pound green beans, trimmed

Preparation

1. Cook the spaghetti per the directions on the package. Drain it.
2. In the meantime, use a large skillet on medium heat, and heat two teaspoons of sesame oil. Add in the pork and sauté for four minutes, stirring occasionally. Add in the bok choy, onions, garlic, soy sauce, pepper, and ginger, and sauté for another three minutes until the pork is cooked through.
3. Meanwhile, use a small skillet (nonstick) to heat olive oil on medium heat. Add in eggs and cook until they

are set (around three minutes). Flip the eggs carefully, and continue to cook for another two minutes. Transfer these to a cutting board and chop them into bite-sized pieces.

4. Next, bring a medium pot of water to boil. Add in the beans and simmer them until they are tender-crisp. Drain the water after three to four minutes.

5. Add the spaghetti, beans, and the remaining teaspoon of sesame oil to the pork mixture. Toss to combine well. Top this with eggs and serve.

Chile Orange Chicken Wings and Ranch Slaw

Prep time: 30 minutes

Duration: 60 minutes

Serves: Four

Nutritional Facts

Serving size: 1/4 of recipe

Calories: 431

Carbohydrate content: 21 grams

Cholesterol content: 85 milligrams

Fat content: 32 grams

Fiber content: 4 grams

Protein content: 15 grams

Saturated fat: 6 grams

Sodium content: 853 milligrams

Sugar content: 9 grams

Monounsaturated fat: 11 grams

Polyunsaturated fat: 14 grams

Ingredients

Wings

- 1 pound split chicken wings, patted dry
- 2 teaspoons of tapioca starch
- 2 tablespoons of orange zest
- 1 teaspoon of chile powder, garlic powder each
- 1/2 teaspoon of salt, smoked paprika, ground cumin each
- 1/4 teaspoon of black pepper

Orange Sauce

- 3/4 cup of fresh orange juice
- 2 tablespoons of tomato paste, unsalted
- 2 tablespoons of coconut aminos
- 2 tablespoons of whole-grain mustard
- 2 teaspoons of tapioca starch
- 1 teaspoon of garlic powder
- 1/2 teaspoon of red pepper flakes
- 1/8 teaspoon of sea salt

Slaw

- 1/2 cup of olive oil mayonnaise
- 1 tablespoon of lemon zest and 2 tablespoons of lemon juice
- 2 tablespoons of chopped chives
- 1 teaspoon of garlic powder
- 1/2 teaspoon of dried dill, black pepper, each
- 1/8 teaspoon of sea salt
- 4 cups of shredded cabbage mix

Preparation

1. Start by lining a baking sheet with foil and place a metal rack on top of foil. Use a large bowl and put in chicken wings. Add the tapioca starch, toss, and coat. In a small bowl, add the remaining ingredients for the wings. Sprinkle over the chicken wings and rub the mixture on the wings. Next, place the wings on the baking rack over the baking sheet. Place the baking sheet with wings in the refrigerator for around eight hours.

2. Preheat the oven to 450 degrees. Place the baking sheet with the wings in the oven and cook for around 20 minutes. Flip the wings and bake for another 20 to 30 minutes.

3. In the meantime, make the sauce. Place a small

saucepan on medium-low heat and whisk together all the sauce ingredients. Bring this mixture to a boil and then reduce the heat to medium low. Allow it to simmer for two minutes or until the sauce begins to thicken. Remove it from heat and set it aside.

4. Transfer the wings to a bowl and drizzle them with a few tablespoons of orange sauce. Toss to coat completely. Reserve the remaining sauce.

5. Prepare the slaw: use a bowl to combine mayonnaise, juice and lemon zest, garlic powder, dill, chives, salt, and pepper. In a large bowl, place the shredded cabbage mix and drizzle the dressing over the top to coat it.

6. Serve the wings with slaw and the reserved orange sauce for dipping.

Seared Sesame Tuna Wraps

Prep time: 10 minutes

Duration: 15 minutes

Serves: Four

Nutritional Facts

Serving size: 1/4 of recipe

Calories: 521

Carbohydrate content: 12 grams

Cholesterol content: 74 milligrams

Fat content: 39 grams

Fiber content: 5 grams

Protein content: 31 grams

Saturated fat: 5 grams

Sodium content: 643 milligrams

Sugar content: 4 grams

Monounsaturated fat: 26 grams

Polyunsaturated fat: 6 grams

Ingredients

- 1/2 cup of avocado oil mayonnaise
- 3 teaspoons of wasabi vinegar
- 1 teaspoon of raw honey
- 3 tablespoons of sesame seeds
- 1 pound tuna belly, pat dry
- 2 tablespoons of avocado oil, divided
- 1/2 teaspoon of sea salt
- 1/4 teaspoon of black pepper
- 6 sheets of nori, unseasoned, cut in half widthwise
- 1 avocado, peeled, pitted, sliced
- 1/2 English cucumber, lengthwise quartered
- 1 carrot cut into matchsticks

Preparation

1. Use a small bowl to mix together wasabi paste, mayonnaise, honey, and vinegar.

2. Put the sesame seeds in a large dish. Rub the tuna with 1/2 of the oil and then season it with salt and pepper. Next, dredge the fish in sesame seeds to coat it.

3. Put a large skillet on medium-high heat, and heat up the remaining 1/2 of the oil. Add in tuna, cook for three to six minutes. Turn it once until it is just seared on the outside. Transfer it to a cutting board and slice it into strips.

4. Arrange the nori sheets on a flat work surface, with the shiny face down. Keep the long end in front of you. Place even amounts of avocado, fish, carrots, and cucumbers at a 45-degree angle. This should be just above the bottom-left corner of every sheet. Drizzle it lightly with wasabi mayo. Roll these into cones and use water to seal the outer seam. Serve with the remainder of the wasabi mayo as a side.

Grilled Mussels Scampi

Prep time: 15 minutes

Duration: 20 minutes

Serves: Four

Nutritional Facts

Serving size: 1/4 of recipe

Calories: 433

Carbohydrate content: 12 grams

Cholesterol content: 133 milligrams

Fat content: 29 grams

Protein content: 31 grams

Saturated fat: 15 grams

Sodium content: 717 milligrams

Sugar content: 1 gram

Monounsaturated fat: 8 grams

Polyunsaturated fat: 2 grams

Ingredients

- 1/2 cup of butter, unsalted, cut in pieces
- 1 small shallot, minced
- 4 cloves of garlic, minced
- 3 tablespoons of fresh parsley
- 1 tablespoon of lemon juice
- 1/2 teaspoon of salt
- 1/4 teaspoon of black pepper
- 4 pounds mussels, debearded and scrubbed
- 8 slices of sourdough bread

Preparation

1. Preheat a grill to medium.

2. In the meantime, using a small saucepan, combine butter, garlic, and shallots. Heat until the butter melts. Allow the mixture to sizzle for a minute before removing it from heat. Add in parsley, lemon juice, and season with salt and pepper. Set this aside.

3. Put the mussels on the grill in a single layer. Work in batches, if required. Cover these and cook until the shells open. This should take around six minutes. Discard the ones that do not open. Transfer the cooked ones into a bowl. Place the bread on the grill and cook until grill marks appear (around one to two minutes each side).

4. Warm up the butter mixture while dividing the mussels among bowls. Drizzle with the butter mixture or serve it as a side. Serve with bread.

Coconut Curry Scallops

Duration: 15 minutes

Serves: Four

Nutritional Facts

Serving size: 1 cup

Calories: 278

Carbohydrate content: 15 grams

Cholesterol content: 51 milligrams

Fat content: 14 grams

Fiber content: 3 grams

Protein content: 27 grams

Saturated fat: 11 grams

Sodium content: 545 milligrams

Sugar content: 5 grams

Monounsaturated fat: 1 gram

Polyunsaturated fat: 1 gram

Ingredients

- 1 tablespoon of coconut oil
- 1 1/2 tablespoons of minced and peeled ginger
- 1 clove of garlic, minced
- 1 tablespoon of curry powder
- 1 tablespoon of ground turmeric
- 1/2 teaspoon of ground cinnamon
- 1 pound bay scallops, rinsed, patted dry (defrosted overnight, if frozen)
- 1 cup of trimmed green beans
- 1 cup of cubed orange bell pepper
- 3/4 cup of full-fat coconut milk
- 1/2 cup of plain yogurt
- 1/2 cup of quartered button mushrooms
- 1/2 lemon, juiced

- 1/4 cup of fresh basil, sliced thinly

Preparation

1. Using a large skillet on medium-high heat, heat the oil. Add in garlic, ginger, curry, cinnamon, and turmeric, and sauté for 30 seconds to a minute until fragrant. Add the scallops, bell pepper, and green beans and sauté for another two to three minutes. Stir occasionally.

2. Stir in the coconut milk, mushrooms, and yogurt. Reduce the heat to medium and allow it to simmer for four minutes. Turn the heat off and add in the lemon juice, and stir. Garnish this with basil.

SAUCES AND DIPS

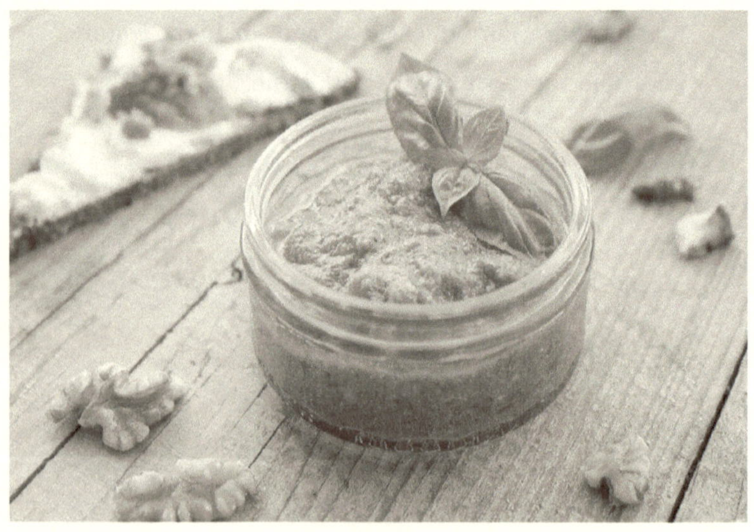

Here are five of my most favorite sauce and dip recipes which are worth trying. They also fit well with the entire diet plan and provide some great taste as well.

THE RECIPES

Mayo Free Ranch Dressing

Prep time: 10 minutes

Duration: 10 minutes

Serves: 10

Nutritional Facts

Serving size: Per 1 gram

Calories: 81

Carbohydrate content: 2.9 grams

Cholesterol content: 20 milligrams

Fat content: 6 grams

Protein content: 3.5 grams

Saturated fat: 3.4 grams

Sodium content: 127 milligrams

Sugar content: 2.1 grams

Ingredients

- 1 cup of plain Greek yogurt
- 1 cup of sour cream
- 1 tablespoon of extra virgin olive oil
- 1/2 cup of milk
- 1 teaspoon of garlic salt
- 2 teaspoons of white wine vinegar

- 1 tablespoon of lemon juice
- 1/4 teaspoon of pepper
- 1/4 cup of chopped scallions
- 1/4 cup of fresh chopped parsley

Preparation

1. Simply mix all the ingredients together until they are smooth. Taste the mixture and add salt and/or pepper to taste. You should refrigerate until it is time to serve.

Homemade Sugar-Free Teriyaki Sauce

Ingredients

- 1 cup of soy sauce (you can also use tamari as a gluten-free option)
- 1 cup of mirin (rice wine)
- 1 to 2 garlic cloves, peeled and crushed
- 1 inch of ginger, cut into three pieces

Preparation

1. Begin by placing all the ingredients in a saucepan. Bring this to a boil and then allow it to simmer for five to ten minutes or until the mixture is down to around one cup.

2. Allow it to cool, scoop out the ginger and garlic, and then refrigerate it.

3. To marinate chicken legs or wings, coat the meat with this sauce and then marinate for one to four hours. When ready, cook at 375 degrees for around 45 minutes.

Homemade Tomato Ketchup

Prep time: 5 minutes

Duration: 25 minutes

Serves: 38 ounces

Nutritional Facts

Serving size: Per ounce

Calories: 15

Carbohydrate content: 2 grams

Sodium content: 102 milligrams

Sugar content: 1 gram

Ingredients

- 28 ounces of tomato puree
- 6 ounces of tomato paste
- 1 tablespoon of olive oil
- 2 cloves of garlic, minced
- 1/4 cup of apple cider vinegar

- 1/4 cup of red wine vinegar
- 1 tablespoon of dried and minced onion
- 1/4 teaspoon of ground cloves
- 1/2 teaspoon of oregano
- 1 teaspoon of salt
- 1/4 cup of granular sweetener

Preparation

1. Add in all the ingredients and blend them using a blender until you have reached the desired consistency.
2. Taste the mixture and adjust the spices or sweetener accordingly
3. Store this in an airtight container and refrigerate it.

Stove Top Cooking

1. Heat up oil and sauté the garlic until it is fragrant.
2. Add in one cup of chopped onions and cook these until softened.
3. Pour the vinegar in, add sweetener of your choice and salt.
4. Bring the mixture to a boil.
5. Add in the tomato puree and the paste.
6. Bring it to another boil.
7. Add in the cloves and the oregano.

8. Cook these until reduced, and the mixture thickens (about 15-20 minutes).

9. Pour this into a blender and blend it until it is smooth.

10. Pour the mixture into a ketchup bottle or a Mason jar.

11. Refrigerate it.

Note: This recipe makes around 30 ounces if made with stove top method. If using a blender, you may get around 38 ounces.

Homemade Salsa

Prep time: 5 minutes

Duration: 5 minutes

Serves: 16

Nutritional Facts

Serving size: 4 ounces

Calories: 31

Carbohydrate content: 5 grams

Fat content: 1 gram

Saturated fat: 2 grams

Sodium contents 148 milligrams

Sugar content: 2 grams

Ingredients

- 28 ounces of whole peeled tomatoes drained
- 20 ounces of diced tomatoes
- 1 cup of chopped onions
- 1 cup of chopped red pepper
- 1 jalapeño pepper (seeds removed), chopped
- 2 cloves of garlic, chopped
- 1/2 cup of cilantro, chopped
- Juice of 1 lime
- 1/2 teaspoon of salt
- 1/2 teaspoon of ground cumin
- 1 tablespoon of olive oil

Preparation

1. Place all of the ingredients into and blend them well using a food processor. Pulse five times if you intend to have chunky salsa or 10 times for a restaurant-style salsa.
2. This recipe will make around five and a half cups of salsa.
3. Keep salsa refrigerated.

Classic Homemade Hummus

Prep time: 1 minute

Duration: 1 minute

Serves: 16

Nutritional Facts

Serving size: Per 1 gram

Calories: 164

Carbohydrate content: 14 grams

Fat content: 11 grams

Protein content: 4 grams

Sodium content: 235 milligrams

Fiber content: 3 grams

Ingredients

- 2 15-ounce cans of chickpeas, drained, rinsed, with around 1/3 cup of juice reserved
- 1/2 a cup of tahini
- 2 cloves of garlic, minced
- 1/2 teaspoon of salt
- 1/2 cup of extra virgin olive oil
- Juice of 2 lemons

Preparation

1. Add in all the ingredients in a food processor or blender.
2. Mix until the desired consistency is achieved.
3. This recipe makes around four cups.
4. Keep it refrigerated.

SNACKS

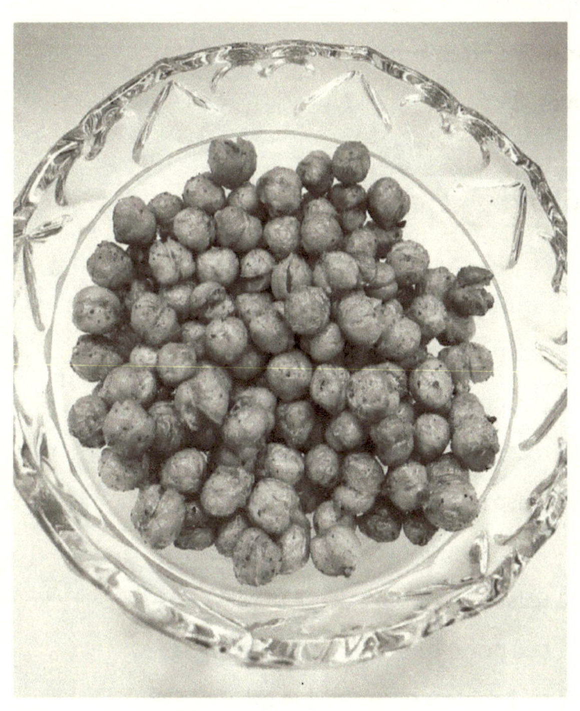

Of course, you do not always have the time to make proper meals. Sometimes, we all need some snacks to fill in the gaps and ensure we continue to feel full, and that is where great snacks come in.

Below, you will find my top five snack recipes of all time.

SNACK TIME RECIPES

Crunchy Roasted Chickpeas

Prep time: 10 minutes

Duration: 50 minutes

Serves: 8

Ingredients

- 1 15-ounce can of chickpeas
- 1/2 teaspoon of ground cumin
- 1/2 teaspoon of smoked paprika
- 1/2 teaspoon of garlic powder
- 1/4 teaspoon of onion powder
- 1/4 teaspoon of ground coriander
- 1/2 teaspoon of sea salt
- 1/4 teaspoon of ground black pepper
- 1/2 to 1 tablespoon of olive oil

Preparation

1. Start by preheating the oven to 400 degrees.
2. Take a baking sheet and lightly spray it with a nonstick spray. Set it aside.
3. Rinse and dry the chickpeas.
4. Use a small bowl to mix together paprika, cumin, sea salt, garlic powder, onion powder, and the pepper. Set this aside.
5. Bake the dried chickpeas in the oven for 15 minutes.
6. Remove chickpeas from the oven and drizzle them with 1/2 tablespoon of olive oil. Stir these to coat evenly. You can add additional oil if needed.
7. Add the spices, and stir.
8. Bake at 400 degrees for another 10 minutes, and then stir.
9. Return them to the oven and bake for five to 10 more minutes, until you have achieved the desired crispiness. Let the chickpeas cool in the oven, leaving the door slightly ajar.

Three-Ingredient Chocolate Cookie

Servings: Approximately 15 cookies

Ingredients

- 2 ripe, large bananas
- 1 cup of gluten-free oats
- Up to 2 tablespoons of unsweetened cacao (to taste)
- Optional add-ons (chocolate chips, chopped nuts, raisins, flax seeds, vanilla, etc.)

Preparation

1. Preheat the oven to 350 degrees. Line a baking sheet with parchment paper.
2. Mash together both bananas in a medium bowl. Mix up to two tablespoons of cacao powder and one cup of oats, and mash until a batter is formed. Remember that the mixture will initially look dry, but on further mixing, it will have a good consistency.
3. Add in the additional add-ins of your choice at this point.
4. Put about 15 clumps of the dough mixture on the baking sheet evenly. Form a cookie shape using your hands.
5. Bake for around 10 to 15 minutes.
6. Serve.

Turmeric Roasted Cashews with Chia

Ingredients

- 2 cups of raw cashew nuts
- 1 tablespoon of chia seeds
- 1/2 teaspoon of ground turmeric
- 1/2 teaspoon of salt
- 1 teaspoon of chili flakes
- 2 teaspoons of dried rosemary
- 1 tablespoon of extra virgin olive oil

Preparation

1. Preheat the oven to 140 degrees.
2. Put the cashew nuts in a large bowl, and add in all the ingredients. Toss well to mix them.
3. Spread the nuts on a rimmed baking tray evenly. Put the tray in the oven and bake these for 10 minutes. Remove from the oven, toss, and spread them evenly. Bake them once again for another 10 minutes until you see a darker shade appearing.
4. Remove them from the oven and let them cool off. You can then store these in a jar for a maximum of two weeks.

Baked Granola Bars

Prep time: 10 minutes

Duration: 35 minutes

Servings: 10-12 bars

Ingredients

- 3/4 cup of gluten-free rolled oats, ground in a flour
- 1 cup of water
- 3/4 cup of pitted Medjool dates
- 1/2 cup of chia seeds
- 1/4 cup of raw sunflower seeds
- 1/4 cup of raw pumpkin seeds
- 1/4cup of dried cranberries, chopped finely
- 1 teaspoon of cinnamon
- 1 teaspoon of pure vanilla extract
- 1/4 teaspoon of sea salt

Preparation

1. Preheat the oven to 325 degrees. Line a square pan with two pieces of parchment paper, one going each way.
2. Use a high-speed blender and add in rolled oats. Blend at the highest speed until it changes into a fine flour form. Add this flour into a large bowl.

3. Add the water and pitted dates in the blender. It is best to allow the dates to soak in the water for 30 minutes, to ease the blending process. Blend until the mixture is very smooth.

4. Add all of the ingredients in the bowl with the flour and stir them together to mix.

5. Scoop the mixture out and into the pan. Spread using spatula evenly.

6. Bake these for 23 to 25 minutes. Once they are firm to the touch, allow them to cool for five minutes. Transfer them to a cooling rack and let them further cool down for 10 minutes. Slice and then enjoy these.

Pecan Date Energy Bites

Prep time: 10 minutes

Duration: 10 minutes

Servings: 15 balls

Ingredients

- 1 cup of pecans (more for topping, if required)
- 1 cup of shredded, unsweetened coconut
- 1/4 cup of almond butter (more for topping, if required)
- 8 to 10 dates

Preparation

1. Use a food processor and process almond butter, dates, pecans, and coconut. Process these until the mixture starts to form a ball and is combined well. If needed, stop and scrape the sides.
2. Remove from the processor and set aside. Using parchment paper, line a baking sheet. Roll the mixture into balls then place these on the baking sheet.
3. Add any additional topping here.
4. Place in the fridge or the freezer to set. Once done, store these in an airtight container within the fridge. Serve as per your needs.

21 DAYS LATER...

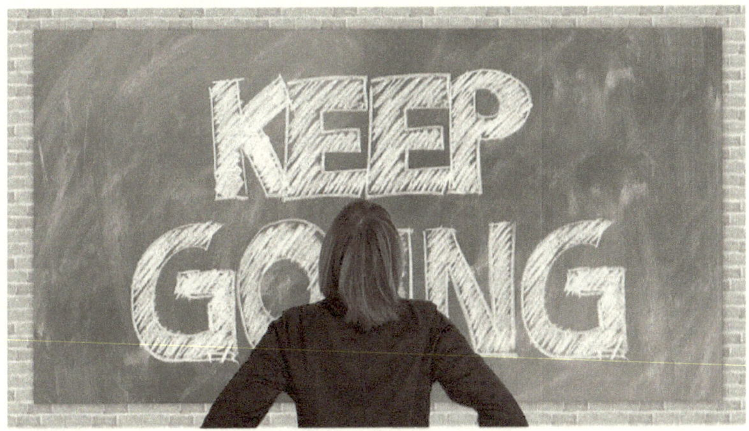

If you start following these recipes and mix them up as you go along, you will not only have some scrumptious meals, but you will also have a significant number of items to choose from. However, the journey is not done.

The first 21 days are a bit tricky, especially after you decide to let go of added sugar. After having fully recovered from the initial symptoms, the next leg of the journey is one that is permanent. A diet is not just something we do for a set period of time and hope that the benefits we gather will last a lifetime. The effort is never ending, which is why the diet you choose is a lifestyle choice; it remains with you for life.

Fortunately, after having gone through 21 days, your body will have grown accustomed to the new changes. It will be ready to welcome more benefits and let go of all those habits that were damaging it. Keeping the momentum going, at least in this case, is far more important than you might imagine.

This chapter does not necessarily present anything you may not already know, but it does offer a brief look into what you can expect after the first 21 days pass. You shouldn't just take my word for it, though. I want you to experience each of these benefits yourself, which will be the true reward.

A COMPLETELY NEW WORLD

We know what GI scores are. All of the above-mentioned recipes provide you with significantly healthy ingredients, all of which fall under the better GI rankings. This means that you do not have to worry about consuming anything that may have a high dose of added sugar or even a higher dose of naturally occurring sugar. All of the recipes above have been carefully selected to ensure that your diet leads you to improve your health while discarding sugar from your daily intake.

Of course, a lot of these recipes may not have ingredients that are readily available within your pantry, which means that you now have a solid excuse to clean out your pantry and make room for healthier ingredients to come in.

After the first 21 days, start experimenting with the recipes. If you come across a new idea, do not be shy to explore it either. As long as you continue to use healthier options, you do not have to worry about sticking to a specific recipe to the letter. You can add or take away things you may or may not like. Even changing one ingredient can often lead to surprising results. Who knows? I may be reading about your recipe someday soon!

It is also a good idea to remember to add fruits after the first 15 days. Some of the recipes above do have fruits, which we are to avoid as they contain fructose, which can often kick in the sugar cravings. After the 21st day, you can start adding a little more fruit to your regular intake. It is tricky (we have our dear food industry to thank for that), but it is not impossible to try and manage your sugar intake. Almost everything we pick up contains added sugar these days.

Live Good, Feel Good

The biggest benefit that you will start experiencing after the 21-day diet will be a clear increase in confidence, morale, and overall health. You will feel better, you will have more energy, and you will feel positive.

They say that a person is what they eat, and since that is the case, it is time to pat yourself on the back for a job well done.

The next step is what makes this change even more interesting: getting to know like-minded people. It greatly helps everyone to know that there are others who have experienced the same journey, and just sharing their accomplishments is a huge morale booster by itself. You may have a lot of people in your vicinity who might have already walked this path. Get to know them, because by doing so, not only are you socializing but you may also end up picking up even better tips and recipes.

The Saga Continues

The real journey begins after the first 21 days. Once you have completed this phase, it is a never-ending struggle to ensure that this becomes your new lifestyle. Make no mistake, even though your body may get used to the new setting, the sight of sugar alone may leave you sweaty and can easily tempt you to break the momentum and find yourself back where you started. You can prevent that by involving more people you know in your social circle, especially those who continue to motivate and inspire you.

The next best thing you can do is to ensure that you always take time out to prepare your meals so they're ready when you need them. This will ensure that you never have a reason to buy premade or precooked meals. Finally, by choosing to stay with this lifestyle, you are letting those massive industries know who the boss really is. While they may continue to prioritize profits over the lives of many, it is up to you, and those like you, to prioritize your own health first.

With that said, we have come to a point where it is time for me to say goodbye and wish you the healthiest of lives ahead. You do not need to feel intimidated anymore. You know everything you need to be successful, and all that remains is for you to act—the reward is yours for the taking!

CONCLUSION

With well over seven billion lives at stake, a number of industries continue to push sugar into the lives of everyone. They do not do this because it helps anyone feel any better: they do it to make these billions of people into addicts and keep them coming for more. The only true winners here are these industries, which continue to count their money, while we are left in the wake of disaster, counting the lives we continue to lose. That comes to an end with a simple change of habits—in comes the sugar-free diet!

When we began this journey, most of us might not have known much about sugar-free diets, except for how hard or expensive they can be, or how they are useless. I am here to tell you otherwise. They are neither expensive, nor are they useless. Yes, they may be hard, but every good thing comes after a struggle.

Sugar-free diets are not exactly 100% sugar free. There is always a trace of sugar that still creeps in, and we actually need that. Our body is designed to work on glucose as fuel. Take that away and it will cease to function. The sugar-free diet actually aims to rid added sugar from the diet. It is this type of sugar that goes on to cause havoc and chaos, not the one that forms naturally.

Throughout this book, we went in great depths about what monosaccharides are, how sugar acts, how added sugar differs, and we even learned a lot about the possible symptoms of sugar addiction that we may be facing. After many pages of science and facts, we finally learned the great recipes. We began with breakfast, headed over to lunch, ended the day with dinner, and we even picked up some recipes for snacks and dips. Finally, we got to look into how life must go on, the great benefit that this diet brings, and how simple techniques like socializing can help keep us from going back to where we started from.

All in all, the journey has been anything but easy, which is why I am extremely proud that you have made it this far. You have everything you need to get started. Twenty-one days later, you may not even need to revisit this book at all, but you will certainly know that you made a wise choice by putting into practice the knowledge you have gained here. It will go on to serve you throughout your life, or at least as long as you decide to keep going with the entire "sugar-free" lifestyle idea.

I would love to know how I was able to help you out, and the only way I can know this is through your feedback. If you found this book helpful, if I was able to provide you with useful knowledge, do write back, and I would love to read what you have to say. In the meantime, I wish you bon voyage and happy trails!

REFERENCES

All photos courtesy of https://pixabay.com/

Avena, N. M., Rada, P., & Hoebel, B. G. (2008). Evidence for sugar addiction: Behavioral and neurochemical effects of intermittent, excessive sugar intake. *Neuroscience & Biobehavioral Reviews, 32*(1), 20–39. https://doi.org/10.1016/j.neubiorev.2007.04.019

Basu, S., Yoffe, P., Hills, N., & Lustig, R. H. (2013). The relationship of sugar to population-level diabetes prevalence: An econometric analysis of repeated cross-sectional data. *PLoS ONE, 8*(2), e57873. https://doi.org/10.1371/journal.pone.0057873

Capritto, A. (2020, May 23). *Is the low-sugar diet the cure-all for health?* Verywell Fit. https://www.verywellfit.com/low-sugar-diet-pros-cons-and-how-it-works-4689214

Clean Eating Magazine. (n.d.). *Clean Eating Magazine*. Clean Eating Magazine. https://www.cleaneatingmag.com/

Guo, X., Park, Y., Freedman, N. D., Sinha, R., Hollenbeck, A. R., Blair, A., & Chen, H. (2014). Sweetened beverages, coffee, and tea and depression risk among older US adults. *PLoS ONE*, *9*(4), e94715. https://doi.org/10.1371/journal.pone.0094715

Health Designs. (2017, October 30). *Natural vs refined sugar: Why the difference matters*. Health Designs. https://www.healthdesigns.net/natural-vs-refined-sugar/

Healy, M. (2015, June 29). *Sugary drinks linked to 25,000 deaths in the U.S. each year*. Latimes.Com; Los Angeles Times. https://www.latimes.com/science/sciencenow/la-sci-sn-sugary-soda-death-toll-20150629-story.html

Johns Hopkins Medicine. (n.d.). Obesity, sugar and heart health. Hopkinsmedicine.Org. https://www.hopkinsmedicine.org/health/wellness-and-prevention/obesity-sugar-and-heart-health

Kaiser Permanente. (2019, January 3). *Sources of glucose | Kaiser Permanente Washington*. Kaiserpermanente.Org. https://wa.kaiserpermanente.org/healthAndWellness/index.jhtml?item=%2Fcommon%2FhealthAndWellness%2Fconditions%2Fdiabetes%2FglucoseSources.html

Kelland, K. (2019, April 4). *One in five deaths worldwide linked to unhealthy diet*. U.S.; Reuters. https://www.reuters.

com/article/us-health-diet/one-in-five-deaths-worldwide-linked-to-unhealthy-diet-idUSKCN1RF2SV

Kubala, J. (2018, June 3). *11 reasons why too much sugar is bad for you*. Healthline. https://www.healthline.com/nutrition/too-much-sugar

Magner, E. (2018, August 10). *What happens when you stop eating sugar? A MD explains*. Well+Good. https://www.wellandgood.com/what-happens-to-your-body-when-you-stop-eating-sugar/

Mayo Clinic. (2018, November 16). *How to add more fiber to your diet*. Mayo Clinic. https://www.mayoclinic.org/healthy-lifestyle/nutrition-and-healthy-eating/in-depth/fiber/art-20043983

National Institute of Health. (2014, October). *Sweet stuff*. NIH News in Health. https://newsinhealth.nih.gov/2014/10/sweet-stuff

New Hampshire Department of Health and Human Services. (n.d.). How much sugar do you eat? You may be surprised! Added sugars. In *dhhs.nh.gov*. https://www.dhhs.nh.gov/dphs/nhp/documents/sugar.pdf

Segal, R. (2019, June). *Choosing healthy fats*. HelpGuide.Org. https://www.helpguide.org/articles/healthy-eating/choosing-healthy-fats.htm

Smith, S. (2019, May 16). *The no-sugar diet plan: Food list & more for getting results*. Onnit Academy. https://www.onnit.com/academy/the-no-sugar-diet-plan/

Villines, Z. (2019, July 4). *What is the glycemic index? Definition, foods, and more*. Www.Medicalnewstoday.Com. https://www.medicalnewstoday.com/articles/325660

Web MD. (n.d.). *What is metabolic syndrome?* WebMD. https://www.webmd.com/heart/metabolic-syndrome/metabolic-syndrome-what-is-it#1

West, H. (2019, April 9). *8 ways food companies hide the sugar content of foods*. Healthline. https://www.healthline.com/nutrition/8-ways-sugar-is-hidden

9 798562 047229